All Women Are Healers

○

A Comprehensive Guide To Natural Healing

By Diane Stein

 **The Crossing Press**
Freedom, California 95019

Note to the Reader:
The information in this book does not constitute
medical advice. Not every suggestion applies to
your particular case. Consult a trusted health
professional if questions arise. Neither the
author nor the publisher take responsibility for
any ill effects which may be produced as a result
of following any suggestions given in this book.
The reader does so at her own risk.

Copyright © 1990 by Diane Stein

Cover illustration by Susan Boulet
Cover design by Betsy Bayley
Typesetting by Claudia L'Amoreaux
Interior illustrations by Melanie Lofland

Printed in the U.S.A.

Library of Congress Cataloging-in-Publication Data

Stein, Diane, 1948-
    All women are healers : a comprehensive guide to natural
healing /
    by Diane Stein
        p.   cm.
    ISBN 0-89594-409-X
    1. Women healers. 2. Mental healing.   I. Title
RZ401.S8116   1990
615.8'52—dc20   89-78396
                                          CIP

All Women
Are Healers

ACKNOWLEDGEMENTS

I would like to thank some of the people who have helped in the research and editing of this book, contributing their time and expertise to bringing accurate healing information to women. I thank Nett Hart and Lee Lanning for their thoughtful comments and for editing yet another of my books. I thank Rebecca Tallman also, for comments and editing and for help with the chapters on vitamins and herbs, and Sidney Spinster for her expertise and editing of the homeopathy chapter. Pam Martin and Denise Messina I thank for reviewing the chapters on polarity balancing, acupressure and applied kinesiology, and for showing me how positive the skills are by using them on me. I thank Russ Osberg and Ron Augustine for general support and caring, and for their input and help as my healing partners.

The generosity and caring of the women at several bookstores has also a been major help in the referencing and locating of materials for this book. Among them, I thank Sally and Beth of Lodestar Books in Birmingham, AL, Harriet and Len of Sign of Aquarius in Pittsburgh, PA, Cheryl and Dana of Goldenseal in Pittsburgh, and the women of Perelandra Books in Eugene, OR. Without their help and generosity this book could not have been written.

For Nett Hart and Lee Lanning
who have edited all my books.

We are all learning to heal, heal ourselves, heal our bodies, heal our common womanspirits. Healing begins in acute attention—attention to our needs and desires, attention to our manifestations. We heal by knowing our state of being, whether we are hot or cold, wet or dry, soothed or irritated, full or empty, sad or content, restless or energetic. We do not need to find cause for this state. By attending to ourselves we can ask 'what do I need to feel whole, well?' We will know the answer. We affirm we can be whole, can have health. We are each ultimately our own healers.

> Nett Hart and Lee Lanning, *Awakening, An Almanac of Lesbian Lore and Vision*, (Minneapolis, Word-Weavers, 1987).

The suppression of female healers by the medical establishment was a political struggle, first in that it is part of the history of sex struggle in general. The status of women as healers has risen and fallen with the status of women. When women healers were attacked they were attacked as *women*; when they fought back they fought back in solidarity with all women.

> Barbara Ehrenreich and Deirdre English, *Witches, Midwives and Nurses: A History of Women Healers*, (Old Westbury, New York, The Feminist Press, 1973).

To administer medicine after an illness begins is . . . like digging a well after becoming thirsty.

> The Chinese *Nei Jing*, 300 BCE.

The term *gynecology*, applied to a branch of patriarchal medicine invented in the nineteenth century as an oppressive/ repressive response and antidote to the first wave of feminism in the United States and Europe, is firmly ensconced in the reversal world.

> Mary Daly, *Websters' First Intergalactic Wickedary of the English Language*, Beacon Press, 1988).

Health is the result of living in harmony with yourself and your environment. Health is to be in sync with life: all the rhythms harmonizing . . . breath with body functions, body functions with life activities, and life activities in rhythm with the cycles of the earth.

> Margot Adair, *Working Inside Out, Tools for Change*, (Berkeley, CA, Wingbow Press, 1984).

I am a woman taking care of myself.
I am a woman who begins the revolution in my own heart,
   who purges from my life the injustices so I can see clearly.
I am a woman unafraid to proceed with what I now know
   knowing as I proceed I will not learn what I could not learn without
I am a woman taking care of myself becoming lean but not hard, separate but
   not apart.
I am a woman who begins the revolution in my own heart.

> Nett Hart and Lee Lanning, *Awakening, An Almanac of Lesbian Lore and Vision*, (Minneapolis, Word Weavers, 1987).

Contents

Introduction

─────────○─────────

Women Heal

Women were the creators of the world, the Goddess-birthgivers, the inventors of positive/peaceful civilization. In every culture, women invented and developed the skills that made survival of the early people possible, from cooking to basketry, gathering to agriculture, domestication of animals to home building. Women first fed themselves and their children by identifying and seeking out wild plants for food and for medicines. In learning how to grow these plants women began agriculture. They developed early tools to make the farming easier, developed basketry and pottery to carry water and to store and cook their harvests in. Women tamed the young of wild animals for wool, milk, pulling plows, carrying heavy objects and for protection, later using animal products for food, clothing and shelters. They developed the art of building structures in various forms—adobe, hides, wood, straw, brick—and the art of making clothes. Primary among their skills and inventions, women began the art and science of healing.

In the time of the early matriarchies, healing and religion were deeply connected and religion was female. Healing began with birth and the act of women giving birth was equated closely with the Goddess' act of creating the world. Every culture had its beginning-of-the-world stories, and the stories were invariably and inevitably birth stories. The Goddess of various and many names arose from chaos to create the earth and universe. From her womb, she formed or gave birth to every species of living thing:

> In the beginning, there was only formless chaos . . . Then chaos settled into form, and that form was the huge Gaea, the deep-breasted one, the earth. (Greece)

Eurynome assumed the form of a dove and laid the Universal Egg on the waves of the sea. She instructed Ophion (the snake also born from her) to coil seven times around this egg until it hatched and split in two. Out tumbled all things that exist. (Greece)

Woyengi (the Mother) molded humans from the Earth while seated with her feet resting on the Creation Stone. (Nigeria)

A woman fell from the upper world. The toad brought her mud from the bottom of the sea. She took it and placed it carefully around the edge of the tortoise's shell. It became the beginning of dry land and of the life upon it. (North America, Huron)

Thou art the mother womb/The one who creates (all). (Babylon)[1]

Through these stories of birth/creation, women saw themselves as images of the birthing Goddess, and midwifery—a matter of species and individual survival—became the foundation of women's healing. Respect for the human mother and the birth process was a form of worshipping the all-creative Goddess, and the relationship of midwife to birthing woman was the first healing partnership.

Along with woman's ability to give birth is her role in nurturing, protecting and training children, and the next foundation of women's healing was in the relationship of mother and child. Until this century, a child that could not be breast-fed died; if the mother was unable to nurse her newborn, a milk-nurse was found. The advent of baby bottles was a late one. Forty-seven percent of the infants raised on bottles died because there was no knowledge of pasteurization until this century.[2] Where the role of the midwife included care of the postpartum mother and her infant, healing extended from the birth itself to the assurance of the child's survival through the mother's nurturance.

In these ideas were the two primary healing roles: that of midwife to birthing woman and of mother to child. These early bases for all the healing arts ensured survival of the tribe and species, and they were matriarchal in attitude. In the case of the midwife to the birthing woman, the midwife helped in the bringing forth of new life. The mother was under her direction but in essence did the work (labor) herself. The midwife, always female, perhaps had children of her own, and perhaps the woman now in labor had once been *her* midwife. The relationship was one of trust and equality, two women participating together to bring life into the world, two women whose roles could be reversed.

In the example of the relationship of mother to child, the mother nursed, nurtured, protected and trained her infant until the child grew up and became independent. In times ahead, when the mother grew old, the now-grown infant or another of her generation could be the one to take care of the aging mother. The daughter could be the one to bring the mother food, help her in her old age, take care of her as her strength waned until her death. Again, there was equality and trust in the mutual roles.

These were the beginnings of healing and medicine: women's needs to care for each other in labor, childhood and old age, to support and maintain each other for the survival of the tribe and species. In medieval Norway, a woman could ask any woman who had already borne a child to help her in her labor and delivery. The penalty for refusal of that request was death, so vital (life-giving) was this relationship. In the early Goddess matriarchies, where to give birth was to become a creation Goddess, such laws were unnecessary. After the child was born and the mother had recovered, the emphasis switched from pregnancy and delivery to keeping the child alive into adulthood. Women, as the caretakers of children, developed into midwives and healers for their own survival and their children's.

A further connection of women with Goddess and with healing came from the menstrual cycle. The matriarchal Goddess was embodied in the earth and the universe, and particularly in the moon. As the earth Goddess, her cycles were the seasons, the growth cycle of agriculture and birth. As the moon Goddess, they were the 28 and 1/2 day menstrual cycle. Women saw their ability for pregnancy and birth as their oneness with the Earth Mother, and their ability to bleed each month as their oneness with the Goddess' lunar cycle. In Greece, the phases of the moon were given Goddess names of Diana for the waxing phase, Selene for the full, and Hecate for the waning period, mirroring the ages of women's lives—youth, maturity and old age.

Observation of women's menstrual/lunar cycles, what was healthy and what was not, and its connection with fertility and control of conception was another aspect that helped to develop women's healing. In early times, when there was no artificial lighting to confuse women's cycles, women menstruated in a regular way, ovulating together on the full moon and menstruating together on the new or dark moon. Women were aware of their natural cycles in synchronicity with the moon's phases and the moon Goddess, and used the lunar cycle to guide conception. Fertility or infertility, conception or contraception, menarche and menopause were women's issues and lunar Goddess issues. The moon in her cycles reflected women's life passages—the new moon as beginnings and birth, the waxing moon from childhood to menarche (first menstruation), the full moon as ovulation and motherhood/fertility, and the waning moon as the celebration of menopause (the ending of menstruation) and aging. Images portraying these ages and life phases as the Three-Form Goddess are worldwide, as are images of the Goddess portrayed as the moon. Issues of women's fertility, mirrored by the lunar month cycle, became issues of women's healing: menarche, menstruation, conception and contraception, fertility, birth and menopause.

From these vital beginnings—woman as earth and moon Goddess creating and nurturing life, participating in the menstrual phases—came women's healing. As woman's knowledge grew and her civilization developed, her knowledge of midwifery, physiology and the techniques of healing grew. The early midwife/healer was a birth coach, pediatrician, gynecologist, nurse, birth control specialist, geriatric physician, psychologist and often veterinarian. She used the tools around her and her developing knowledge of them, passed from mother to daughter, of herbs, bodywork, gemstones, reflexology, touch healing, nutrition and guided meditation to make women's birth experiences easier and to reduce disease and disease mortality rates of newborns, children, adults, birthing mothers and elders. She had the methods and knowledge to control fertility. This was the beginning of science and the beginning of medicine.

Then the matriarchies ended. Work by feminist archeologists Merlin Stone and Marija Gimbutas[3] trace the ending of matriarchy to Nordic, nomadic tribes from what are now Scandanavia and the Russian Steppes moving southward, beginning about 15,000 years ago. These were patriarchal peoples, male-dominated cultures based on the breeding of animals and women. They moved south for unknown reasons—worsening climates, hunger, need for grazing lands. Theirs was a warlike culture using the wheel, chariot and domesticated horse, as well as spears and other weapons—the weaponless and peaceful matriarchies could not withstand them. By 3000 BCE, these tribes took over, destroying earlier civilizations, submerging women and matriarchal cultures, and substituting their male gods for the Goddess. They moved as far south as India and central Africa and as far west as Ireland and Wales, leaving death, devastation and countless refugees behind them.

These were the beginnings of modern culture as we know it. Descendents of these patriarchal tribes became the 'cradle of civilization' cultures of the middle east, the early judaic tribes, and eventually evolved into christianity and islam. With them came patriarchal male-dominance, devaluing women and every aspect of women's Being, denying the life force, the life cycle, and the birthing creation Goddess. Creation was stripped of its female and birth roots, substituting Adam as the first male ancestor, created by a motherless god from dust. With the submergence of Goddess came the submergence of women as civilizers and healers. Cultural growth all but stopped, and civilization regressed drastically for several thousand years.

Many women remembered the Goddess, however, and her worship went underground. The village midwife remained as the primary healer and caregiver of each region and she was often the village high priestess as well. The Goddess religion survived, hidden, despite devastating persecution from patriarchal tribes, governments and male religious forces. In the burnings of the ancient matriarchal libraries before the tenth century, in the decline of the great African and Egyptian trading empires, in the European witch burnings of the thirteenth through seventeenth centuries, and in the christianization of North and South America, much healing knowledge, and knowledge of all facets of women's civilization was lost.

Men first began to enter healing in Europe when the christian church's misogyny increased against woman healers in the fifth to tenth centuries. They entered, organized and controlled what had been a women's skill, and purged women from it. This was the beginning of medicine. Women were outlawed from the practice of healing and later from midwifery, initially by the requirement of a college education to practice medicine. The church-run colleges (and most lower schools) were open only to upper class men. Colleges of that time taught charms and incantations but very little science, while women held real knowledge learned by apprenticeship, oral tradition and experience.

Women who were trained in healing in the old ways, usually the only ones providing medical care for their villages, were burned at the stake for being successful healers. They were seen as competition to the new male doctors who studied philosophy instead of healing. However, since men saw women as the church did, as evil and unclean, they refused to handle deliveries. Midwifery remained in the hands of women until the French male invention of obstetrical forceps in the seventeenth to eighteenth centuries. Only until then and after the loss of women healers to the Inquisition, did men enter and begin to dominate the field of childbirth.

Despite their persecution of women healers, early male doctors knew far less than the women. Practical healing skills remained in women's hands for many more years.

The wise woman, or witch, had a host of remedies which had been tested in years of use. Many of the herbal remedies developed by witches still have their place in modern pharmacology. They had pain killers, digestive aids and anti-inflammatory agents. They used ergot for the pain of labor at a time when the Church held that pain in labor was the Lord's just punishment for Eve's original sin . . . Digitalis is said to have been discovered by an English Witch.

The witch-healer's methods were as great a threat (to the Catholic Church, if not the Protestant), as her results, for the witch was an empiricist; she relied on her senses rather than on faith or doctrine, she believed in trial and error, cause and effect. Her attitude was not religiously passive, but actively inquiring. She trusted her ability to find ways to deal with disease, pregnancy and childbirth—whether through medications or charms. In short her magic was the science of the time.[4]

The witch hunts eliminated the competition from women who had greater knowledge and a more successful rate of healing. It was a political 'final solution' to put men in control of women and of healing. With nine million women dead by the end of the Inquisition, the campaign all but succeeded, sometimes leaving only one woman alive in a village. The few women midwives and healers remaining by the eighteenth century were ridiculed and discredited for their knowledge, as male doctors took over their practices. These early doctors continued to have less knowledge than the healers and far more failures. Unlike the women healers, their services were restricted to those who could afford to pay, leaving many without health care at all.

The legacy of that takeover is still with us, still seen in medicine's repression of holistic health, and women are still the major sufferers in patriarchal medicine. The early reverence of women as images of the creation Goddess is gone, and also gone is the awareness of women as inventors of both healing and peaceful civilization. The judeo-christian and other patriarchal religions' view of women is that women are unclean and "vessels of original sin." Without the Goddess, there is no connection with the earth and respect for natural cycles, but rather a determination to dominate and subdue women and nature. Science has developed, and so has technology, but only the discovery (practiced by the midwives early on) of sanitation has reduced some diseases and lengthened life. Many medical advancements are dehumanizing, frightening and punishing, yet have not decreased mortality rates or raised the quality of life for anyone, (and particularly not for women of color). A woman entering a hospital for childbirth, surgery or even observation/testing has a great risk of becoming sicker or not surviving.

> The technical effectiveness of medicine is very limited. Hospitals could release 85% of their patients without harming them from a strictly medical point of view.[5]

> One out of five patients admitted to a typical research hospital acquires an iatrogenic (doctor caused) disease, sometimes trivial, usually requiring special treatment, and in one case out of thirty leading to death . . . Amazingly, one in ten comes from diagnostic procedures.

> Medications in hospitals alone kill between 60,000 and 140,000 Americans a year and make 3.5 million others more or less seriously ill.

> More than half the surgery performed in this country is unnecessary.

> In 1976 there was a doctor strike in Los Angeles over malpractice rates . . . There was " an almost steady decline in death rates during the doctor slowdown, followed by an abrupt leap upward (from 14 to 26 deaths per 100,000) in the very first week that surgery as usual was resumed."[6]

> According to a nurse on the obstetrical team of a large teaching hospital in New York City, the rate of C-sections (Caesarean births) for one month in 1974 was an unbelievable 50 percent.[7]

> The rate of infant mortality was much higher in America than in fifteen other developed countries in the world . . ." We estimate that between 45,000 and 50,000 babies die unnecessarily" (each year) in the United States " because of inadequate care."[8]

> One study done on comparable populations who chose prepared home birth as opposed to hospital birth found that the infant death rates were about the same for both groups, but that the hospital babies suffered thirty times the number of birth injuries (primarily from the use of forceps), four times as many infections, and 3.7 times as many resuscitations (primarily because of the large proportion of hospital births during which the mother is sedated).[9]

> In many regions of the United States more than 40 percent of the hysterectomies and oophorectomies (removal of uterus and ovaries) have involved removal of *normal* organs.[10]

Women are doctors' direct victims at times of hospital births, where delivery is managed mechanically as a disease process. Over half of surgical births (C-sections or Caesareans) and hysterectomies (surgical removals of women's uterus and/or ovaries) are unnecessary. There is no greater survival rate in breast cancer with radical mastectomies, but thousands of breast removals are performed on women, especially on Black women, each year. Women are a larger percentage of psychiatric patients than men, and "are prescribed more than twice the amount of drugs than are men, for the same psychological symptoms."[11] In general, women see doctors more often than men do and are admitted into hospitals in greater proportions than are men. These are the results of the loss of the women healers, the loss of a Goddess society that respects women and the life force, and some of the reasons for a renaissance in women's healing today.

The loss of the Goddess, the devaluing of birth and life in modern patriarchal society, has other implications that affect women's health. Women in the matriarchies gathered plants and grains for food or grew them, and later in time ate the flesh and milk of animals they organically raised. Food production in the patriarchy has become a dehumanized big industry. Male determination to dominate and subdue the Earth Goddess has resulted in depleted soils and malnourished crops that have little resistance to insects or plant diseases. Chemical fertilizers and insecticides literally poison crops, and the malnourished, chemical-ridden plants are what women depend upon for food. Food animals are fed these inadequate crops, plus hormones and antibiotics to artificially fatten them, and again these are passed on to meat-eating women. The refining process that creates white rice, white sugar and white flour removes most of the nutritive value. Their use is pervasive. White sugar and the overuse of salt are literally poisons of modern society. Food is loaded with salt, to preserve it and to add flavor because the denatured food is tasteless. Fruits and vegetables are picked half-ripe and shipped thousands of miles to supermarkets. It may be weeks or months between harvest and eating. And the newest bright idea of the patriarchy is irradiation of grains, meats, spices, fish, fruits and vegetables to prolong shelf life.

Is it any wonder that cancer, high blood pressure, heart disease, strokes and a variety of other degenerative dis-eases unknown in 1900 are epidemic today? Instead of the clear flowing rivers and underground water sources of the matriarchies, modern water is a dumping place for radioactive and factory-toxic wastes, 'cleaned' for drinking by other toxic chemicals. The air is filled with carbon monoxide from automobiles and industrial and nuclear pollutants and wastes. We don't know how to dispose of radioactive contaminants, or even our household garbage. Tobacco, alcohol and drug abuse (prescribed and recreational) are further pollutants and killers of the individual and environment. Poverty and hunger kill more people today than in any other time in known history. Nuclear war is a constant threat.

In this clear and present danger of a world created by men without the influence of Goddess/women, the need for the return of women healers is vital (life-giving) and obvious. Women are a voice of sense and compassion in the face of increasing technology, mechanization, invasion, and dehumanization of the male way of doing things, from medicine to pollution to processing food, to politics and war. In the threat of patriarchy, the woman healer of the eighteenth century stood as a last reminder of the Goddess and of a matriarchal order that valued women's bodies and birth. The witch/midwife/healer, then and now, was and is

> a woman and not ashamed of it. She appeared to be a part of an organized underground of peasant women. And she was a healer whose practice was based on empirical study. In the face of the repressive fatalism of Christianity, she held out the hope of change in the world.[12]

Today the woman healer holds out the same hope in an even more repressive and complex world. The same Goddess-worshipping, woman-affirming female healers who were the originators and developers of peaceful matriarchal civilization and healing are the hope of the healing/medical profession, of women and our world.

The renaissance/rebirth of women healers is in progress, a trend begun in the 1960s with the beginnings of feminism and return of the Goddess religion. In the early sixties, Black leaders and the hippie and peacenik counterculture engineered the civil rights and anti-war movements. Increasingly influenced by women and women's values, they held a doctrine of love and respect, peace, anti-racism and back-to-nature individualism. They opposed competition, war, money worship, conformity, divisions between the races, and dehumanizing mechanization. At the verge of feminist consciousness, women explored healing techniques and communal societies within this liberal, activist atmosphere for the first time in centuries. They rediscovered ecology, women's handicraft arts, Eastern religions, nonviolence and self-sufficient living and discovered women's rights. Midwifery reemerged as a strong force during the sixties' back-to-land movement, along with massage, yoga, herbs, naturopathy and touch therapies.

These women were the founders of the current women's movement, which in turn was the springboard for the rebirth of the Goddess by radical feminists in the 1970s. Every study of Goddess religion and witchcraft led back to healing, and many women followed where it led. Increasing numbers of women recognized witchcraft as a living alternative to misogynist patriarchal religions and a logical outgrowth of feminist philosophy. Increasing numbers of women also saw alternative healing as a way to regain their identities and bodies under patriarchal medicine. With the great expansion of Goddess into women's lives in the 1980s, the study of healing continues to increase. Learning from books, workshops, at the women's cultural festivals, in public and private circles and study groups, and by self-experimentation, women are reclaiming both Goddess and life-affirming values, and the sciences and arts of women's healing. Using these as an affirmation of women and the life force, of Goddess and Goddess-within, women are reclaiming their power as healers for the benefit of all.

This alternative healing movement has many facets. Women are going back to ancient techniques of herbs and touch healing, to oriental traditions of acupuncture, shiatsu, polarity and reflexology. They are working with newer ideas, such as vitamins, homeopathy and flower remedies. Women are developing muscle testing and pendulum work, and reclaiming and extending work with laying on of stones, crystal patterns, crystals and gemstones. Women are taking the old methods and experimenting with them, broadening, developing and refining them. As in the past, this is a lay-women's movement of skilled practitioners with increasing interest by women chiropractors and a few medical professionals.

By the study, experimentation and practice of natural healing, women are changing and charting the future of health care. Despite heavy resistance or lack of recognition from patriarchal medicine, they are nevertheless making positive changes that will continue and increase. Women's emphasis on one-to-one work practiced in mutual agreement and participation is very different from mechanized and big-money medicine, and has results and successes far beyond expectations. The emphasis on self-healing returns health care to the consumer, to women's lives and bodies, for the first time in centuries. The medical system cannot control a movement held in the hands of women, though it may try. Women are taking control again of healing, our daughter-right, for the first time since the matriarchies and the Inquisition.

Along with the methods, women are reclaiming the peaceful, cooperative, earth and life-affirming attitudes that made the matriarchies the originators of human civilization. Women healers are women activists, fighting racism and hunger, nuclear waste and nuclear war, and the destruction/pollution of water, air, soil and the food chain. They work to end the abuses that threaten women, threaten life and that threaten the Goddess planet. They work to end sexism and misogyny and return the pride, strength, self-love and independence of Goddess/women. For the first time since patriarchal hordes destroyed women's culture, there is hope for women and the survival of the planet.

Each of the ten chapters in this book explores one of the many ways of women's healing, with as much teaching-to-do-it as is possible in each chapter. Midwifery is not included, though it is the root of women's healing. It deserves a book (many books) of its own. This book is a continuation of the material in *The Women's Book of Healing*,[13] and does not repeat (but may overlap) the material and teaching of that book. This volume includes information on other healing techniques not covered in *The Women's Book of Healing*: laying on of stones, Reiki, polarity balancing, Chinese medicine and acupressure, reflexology, muscle testing and pendulum work, applied kinesiology, vitamins, herbs, homeopathy, flower essences and gemstone elixirs.

The reason for this book is to teach women to be healers, to take the initiative of healing away from the medical system as much as possible by preventing dis-ease from becoming serious illness. This is to strengthen, reclaim and affirm the Goddess-ancient practice of women's healing and self-healing.

New moon in Taurus
April 16, 9988

NOTES

1. Judy Chicago, *The Birth Project*, (New York, Doubleday and Co., 1985), pp. 11, 92, 106. For further creation stories, see Merlin Stone, *Ancient Mirrors of Womanhood*, (Boston, Beacon Press, 1984), and Diane Stein, *The Women's Spirituality Book*, (St. Paul, Llewellyn Publications, 1987).

2. Lina G. Straus, *Diseases In Milk*, (New York, E.P. Dutton Co., 1917), pp. 51, 90–91.

3. Marija Gimbutas, *The Goddesses and Gods of Old Europe*, (Berkeley and Los Angeles, University of California Press, 1974 and 1982), and Merlin Stone, *When God Was A Woman*, (New York, Harcourt, Brace, Jovanovich, 1976).

4. Barbara Ehrenreich and Deirdre English, *Witches, Midwives and Nurses, A History of Women Healers*, (Old Westbury, NY, The Feminist Press, 1973), p. 14.

5. Margot Adair, *Working Inside Out, Tools for Change*, (Berkeley, CA, Wingbow Press, 1984), p. 159.

6. *Ibid.*, pp. 158–159. These are quotes from a variety of sources.

7. Suzanne Arms, *Immaculate Deception* , (New York, Bantam Books, 1975), p. 115.

8. *Ibid.*, pp. 43–44.

9. Judy Chicago, *The Birth Project*, p. 196.

10. Barbara Seaman and Gideon Seaman, MD, *Women and the Crisis in Sex Hormones*, (New York, Rawson Associates Publishers, Inc., 1977), p. 308.

11. Muriel Nellis, *The Female Fix*, (Boston, Houghton Mifflin Co., 1980), p. 7.

12. Barbara Ehrenreich and Deirdre English, *Witches, Midwives and Nurses*, p. 15.

13. Diane Stein, *The Women's Book of Healing*, (St. Paul, Llewellyn Publications, 1987).

Chapter One

———————◯———————

Laying On of
Stones and Crystal Patterns

Laying on of stones and gemstone crystal patterns are both the newest and the oldest of women's healing techniques. An outgrowth of Goddess women's intense interest in crystals and gemstones in the past ten years, healing work with stones reaches back into the herstory of every culture. Quartz crystal composes fully a third of the physical makeup of Goddess Earth, and gemstones and crystals are available in some form everywhere. They were known and used for healing in Native America, South America, Africa, Europe and Egypt, and were a highly developed art in ancient India.

Going back further than herstory, the legends and stories of Atlantis, an ancient culture destroyed by earth changes thousands of years ago, are filled with both positive and negative uses of clear quartz crystal. The continent of Atlantis was a highly developed technological civilization with correspondences in its technology and problems to modern western society. Their major source of energy was based on crystal technology, and their healing was powered by crystal and gemstone use beyond current knowledge. Enough information about healing work in Atlantis remains to consider this fabulous, highly developed culture the beginning of gemstone and crystal healing on earth.

A number of women today are bringing to light crystal and gemstone information by psychic means, channeling or automatic writing of directed information. In this method, women in the meditative state allow non-conscious information to be given to them, and they repeat it verbally or write it as it's given. An increasing number of women are linking with this psychic source of powerful information and are channeling material on healing and crystal work stored from Atlantis. Putting the material to experiment and use, they find much of it to be highly valuable. By applying and teaching the information, and by further experimentation, women are developing and increasing modern knowledge of gemstone healing.[1]

Many women believe that a large number of souls who were alive at the height or destruction of Atlantean civilization are in re-incarnation now. Women in past life regression work report the knowledge of lifetimes in Atlantis, or in ancient Egypt soon after, where much of Atlantean learning was preserved from extinction. Many of these women are crystal and gemstone workers today, some drawing from an intuitive source barely remembered or totally unremembered, which nevertheless gives them information when they need it for healing. Much of the crystal and gemstone informa-tion available to women has been given to us quickly in these ways, in a major burst of new and detailed healing knowledge unknown just a few years ago.

The reasons for the sudden gift of crystal and gemstone tech-nology and healing can be speculated. That women returning to Goddess worship and seeking healing methods are ready in their development to use it and that the present need is great is one idea. That women have reached the psychic sensitivity required to re-ceive the information is another possible reason, along with the readiness of supplies of gemstones now available to work with. Other speculations are that the west is reaching a crisis, as Atlantis once did in its long-buried past. We are at a point of deciding to use our technologies for the betterment of life and surviving, or of using our technologies in negative ways and being destroyed by them. Atlantis was believed to have been destroyed by its negative use of crystal technology to oppress others. Many souls who witnessed this choice in Atlantis are reincarnated on earth now, working to prevent another major destruction of a technological empire, hop-ing to assure a positive and life-affirming world. Women healers are an important part of the choice for life-affirming values with their insistence on real values above technology-for-its-own-sake and their insistence on cleaning up the earth and on healing themselves and correcting current abuses.

Laying on of stones is a method that survived Atlantis and the matriarchies' destruction. In more recent herstory than Atlantis, the Egyptian Pharaoh Queens, early queen-healers like Mentuhetop (2300 BCE) and Cleopatra (69–30 BCE)[2] worked extensively with colored stones in healing patterns. Egyptian healing was respected in the Middle East and Africa, and healers from several nations came to Egypt to learn methods from these women. The learning was spread by students to the Mediterranean, and later from

Greece to Europe. India was also known as a healing center, claiming with Egypt its invention of various healing skills including gemstone work. Work with colored gemstones and crystals was highly developed in India, probably from matriarchal times. In Native America, shamans and medicine women of a number of tribes carried crystals in their medicine pouches and used crystal patterns, and turquoise was used extensively on various parts of the body in the North American Southwest.

In Africa, the foremothers of the West African Market Women were revered as sailors and explorers. Black women sailors may have been the ancient Phoenician traders who travelled the world as far as the Americas and the Orient, long before Columbus. From their stops in Egypt and Greece, gemstone work would have been known to these women, and their travels carried knowledge throughout the world. Striking similarities between the Indian Goddess Sarasvati, the Chinese Goddess Kwan Yin and the South American Goddess Chalchiuhtlique indicate that the ancient cultures had knowledge of each other or a common origin such as Atlantis. The Goddesses are drawn much alike in art, and both Kwan Yin and Chalchiuhtlique are represented by jade, an all-healing gemstone of great power. By the similarities, including gemstone knowledge, it is speculated that world communication may have existed long before the modern day, and that the world was once connected by the Phoenician women sailors. Only speculation is now possible, as that communication and herstory are lost, destroyed by the cataclysms that sank Atlantis or the chaos that ended the matriarchies. The evidence, however legendary, is intriguing and, even lacking stronger proof, is as valid as what men have written about women's past.

Whether crystal work and laying on of stones is from Atlantis, from the ancient women's matriarchies, or is something totally new is less important than its use and success by women today. Information is growing rapidly in this remembered field, and is being transmitted to women for immediate use. Along with its ability to release physical dis-ease, laying on of stones has power in working with the emotional sources that cause much physical illness. By use of crystals and gemstones, and particularly by laying on of stones, women release the emotional abuses of patriarchy from their Being, work through issues, and reaffirm their Goddess-within self love. This type of healing is important, as physical manifestation of dis-ease (lack of ease) is a reflection of the nonphysical body from these unseen levels, which are known worldwide.

Where the medical system treats women from physical symptoms only, women's healing works with the physical by way of causes, through working with the unseen psychic layers. Science has agreed by now that the body is surrounded by an electrical field, and healers call that energy the aura. The aura is composed, in eight levels of energy or light, of four unseen bodies that surround and effect the physical body.[3] In esoteric thought, this is where the soul or Being is located, and is also where the physical body's health and growth are directed from.

Some background on the levels and chakras is in order here. The first, closest to physical, of the four bodies is called the **etheric double**. This is basically an energy twin of women's physical body, a reddish-black line of vibrating light that surrounds and follows the body's contours. Also called the physical body aura, this energy twin directs women's states of health. An illness or dis-ease appears first at this level and can be released from it before manifesting as physical pain. The chakras, eight major (and many minor) energy centers that are activated directly in laying on of stones, are located on the etheric double body.

Next to the etheric double, moving outward from the skin, is the **emotional body**. As its name suggests, this energy layer generates emotions, transmitting them through the etheric double to the physical body. Emotions are highly important to women's health. Everyone has had the experience of being upset by her boss, her mate or screaming child and developing a headache or queasy stomach. When a woman is emotionally calm and stable, her health gets better. Louise Hay reveals in her work an emotional source for virtually every physical dis-ease.

Emotions can be transient things and also can be stored. Unreleased anger turns inward to cause physical illness, and is the basic cause of cancer, ulcers, headaches, migraines and arthritis. Unprocessed emotions remain in the emotional body, in the subconscious, to surface in negative ways later that effect health. A major part of women's healing, and particularly laying on of stones, is its use to release blocked emotions, thereby releasing physical dis-ease. In clearing the emotional body of held-in pain, fear and emotional issues, women move closer to well-being. In a society where release of anger is often unsafe or has negative consequences, this role of gemstone healing is especially important.

The third of the aura bodies, comprised of two levels, is the **mental body**. This unseen layer contains the rational and imaginative mind as the lower and higher mental body levels. Rational thinking, the lower mental body, is where most of us live in daily life. It's the analytical, concrete mind, the part of women's Being that reads the newspaper and adds up grocery bills. In this place, women make choices that create conscious ideas, and these ideas transmitted through the emotional body and the etheric double become physically real. At the next level, the rational mind is influenced by imagination (the higher mental body), where thoughts create not what is, but what may be.

In women's healing, the mind and imagination are important tools, with the ability to generate health or dis-ease. Take this example: a woman examining her breasts discovers a small lump. Using her mind and imagination she can do two things while waiting for the biopsy; she can imagine that the lump is benign, as 80 percent of breast lumps are, or she can create for herself the scenario of dying of breast cancer. The trick and the danger here is that often what a woman imagines becomes real. In imagining disaster, the woman causes the image to be picked up and accepted in her rational, lower mind level, from which point the emotions take over with total fear. The emotions in turn pass that fear onto the etheric double, with a good chance of making the negative image happen. If the woman refuses this image, choosing instead her faith that the lump is benign, she transmits *that* image and increases her chances that the lump is harmless.

Taking it a step further, the woman who affirms the lump is harmless can create an image to tell her physical body what to do. If she imagines the lump in her breast shrinking until it dissolves, chances are that by the time she reaches her doctor, the lump will be gone. This is the basis of psychic healing, this use of the mental body levels. Medicine and healing go together here, along with women's intuition. Women often 'know' before the biopsy whether the lump is malignant or benign.

The fourth of women's unseen bodies is the **spiritual body**, comprised of three layers with physical coordinates and one beyond them. These layers, called the lower, middle and higher spiritual bodies and the transpersonal point, are the means of transmitting Goddess-within through women's Being. The more closely a woman can accept herself as part of Goddess and be open to that, the more healing power she is able to transmit through this spiritual body to the mental, emotional and etheric levels and into the physical Being. This is the place of becoming a channel for healing energy or information, for yourself or others, whether drawn from Atlantis, from the higher self, the subconscious, or from Goddess-within.

In this very brief description of the four bodies, make note of the following color coordinates. They are the basis for laying on of stones, gemstone and crystal work, color therapy and other forms of women's healing.

Etheric Double	Black and Red	
Emotional Body	Orange	
Mental Body	Yellow	(Lower mental)
	Green	(Higher Mental)
Spiritual Body	Blue or Aqua	(Lower Spiritual)
	Indigo	(Middle Spiritual)
	Violet	(Higher Spiritual)
	Clear or Colorless	(Transpersonal Point)

The next set of important information involves the chakras, which are a series of eight energy vortices on the etheric double. Laying on of stones works directly with these centers, using gemstones on each chakra to transmit color and light through the four energy bodies. Each chakra has its location on the physical body and a series of attributes and healing uses. Though laying on of stones can be done to energize or heal one chakra only, most layouts work with all the centers to bring the whole woman into balance. The chakras correspond to the levels of the aura, to the four bodies, and to the colors of the aura layers. The colors are the spectrum rainbow, ranging from black to clear/colorless, with seven colors in between.

The **root center** is located at the vagina. Its colors are black and red. Black stones are sometimes placed at the feet, as well as actually on the root center to connect women with the earth. Black is the color of the earth and the inside of the womb. When a woman needs root center calming and grounding or has issues with anxiety, unconnectedness, breaking addictions and habits, fear or pain, her healing color and stones are black. Other black gemstone uses are for colitis, diarrhea, recovery from abortion or miscarriage, difficult menopause or menstruation, and the emotional inability to move forward. Black also corresponds with death, past lives, karma and reincarnation.

Red is the traditional activating color of the root chakra, as the manifestation side of the womb. Its correspondences are life and death, fertility, red blood and physical survival. Red root center issues include: bringing on menstruation, uterine healing, life force energy and vitality, red blood cells, blood circulation, getting pregnant, menarche, increasing menstrual flow, warmth, raising depression, AIDS, leukemia, cancer and constipation. Red stones stimulate the root center while black ones calm and stabilize it. The colors match the etheric double that mirrors the physical body.

Orange is the color of the emotional body level and the chakra is located on the lower abdomen, between the pubic bone and the navel. The **belly chakra** is emotions, particularly stored old ones and first impressions. It's the ovaries in women and the spleen in men, the location of sexuality issues, as well as overlapping the root center in matters of fertility and menstruation. Orange activates the center, while brown and orange/brown gemstones calm and balance it. Women with asthma, allergies, epilepsy, coughs, kidney dis-ease and arthritis work with this chakra, along with issues of pre-orgasm, sexual reopening after painful relationships, ovarian cysts and menstrual pain.

The mental body contains two chakras, the solar plexus and the heart (lower and higher mental bodies). The **solar plexus** is located just above the navel, with its traditional color yellow. Corresponding with the rational mind, the solar plexus works with healing issues of assimilation. These include the intake and distribution of nutrition, ideas, energy and psychic impressions. Yellow activates the center, while yellow-green gemstones balance it, for such healing issues as diabetes, hypoglycemia, eating disorders, digestive upsets, ulcers, urinary infections, apathy, tiredness, increasing mental alertness, raising depression, willpower and visualization.

The imaginative level of the mental body is located at the **heart chakra**, a center located under the breastbone, between the breasts. Heart center issues are especially caused by patriarchal society, literally dealing with broken hearts (heart dis-ease), thymus/immune system strengthening, circulation, infections, loneliness, love, self-image, trust, and recovery from abused childhoods or relationships. The colors here, both balancers, are rose and green, with green traditional. Major issues of the heart center are giving and receiving love, not in a sexual (emotional body/orange) way but in a universal, compassionate way. Heart center gemstones also stimulate the imagination, the child within the woman.

The spiritual body has three chakras, plus the transpersonal point that is beyond the physical entirely. The lower spiritual body chakra is the **throat center**, located in the hollow of the throat. Traditional color is light blue, but aqua (a combination of blue and heart center green) is prominent in the gemstones. The throat directs communication and expression, as well as creativity of all sorts. Its healing uses include sore throats, laryngitis, the voice, pain, inflammations and swellings, burns, headaches, migraines, choking, artist's block, rape and incest recovery, and hearing. Women are taught to hold in their expressions of anger, pain and outrage at the system. Anger internalized is the cause of most throat center healing issues. Anger is also the source of more dis-eases than any other emotion, but used in positive ways is also a source of needed change and release.

The middle spiritual level is located at the brow or **third eye**, and its color is indigo. An alternate color in gemstones is opaque white. Healing uses for this chakra include endocrine balancing, menstrual cycle regulation, the eyes and senses, multiple sclerosis, headaches, mental and nervous disorders, degenerative dis-eases, white blood cells, the lymphatic/immune system, decreasing menstrual flows, colds, flu, pneumonia, psychic development, clairvoyance and internal healing. The center is located over the pituitary gland, the body's major hormone balancer, and is women's power of intuition and knowing.

Violet is the color of the **crown chakra**, the higher spiritual body level. This center, located just past the top of the head, is the place where a baby's fontanelle is open at birth, and is women's connection with Goddess. Violet gemstones work with this chakra for degenerative dis-eases, vision, lymphatic/immunity, stress disorders, headaches, insomnia, white blood cells, anxiety, mental and nervous issues, tumors, strokes, peace of mind and any issues of the head or brain.

Completely beyond the physical body, the **transpersonal point** is several inches above the crown. Whole aura healing is drawn from this chakra, using primarily clear quartz crystal as its gemstone. Clear stones are the only ones used for unifying, clearing and purifying the entire energy field of the body, rather than one specific chakra. The transpersonal point is the place of Goddess and Goddess-within, the source for channeling healing knowledge and energy through all the centers.

Gemstone colors for the eight major chakras are as follows:

Chakra	Activating Color	Balancing Color	Complementary/ Opposite Color
Root	Red	Black	Green
Belly	Orange	Brown	Blue
Solar Plexus	Yellow	Yellow-Green	Violet
Heart	Green	Rose	Red
Throat	Blue	Aqua	Orange
Third Eye	Indigo	White	Orange
Crown	Violet	White	Yellow

Transpersonal
Point   Clear   Clear   Clear

Laying on of stones translates the colors of the chakras and
four bodies into gemstone energies, and any number of stones with
that center's colors are useful for it. Activating and balancing colors
are used most often. In doing a healing, the woman being healed lies
flat on a floor or table and stones for each chakra are placed on her
body's chakra centers. The gemstones can be in any form—rough,
tumbled, cut and polished, or faceted—as long as they are comfortably light pieces. A variety of gemstones can be used for each
chakra, or one type of gemstone on each center. One or many pieces
can be set on each chakra, and where several are used, beautiful
stone patterns evolve in placing them.

The woman being healed and the healer work together. If a
stone feels uncomfortable to either woman, it isn't used. Once a
stone is placed, if the woman being healed chooses to have it moved
or removed, the healer obliges. If the woman wants it on a chakra
where its color doesn't match, that's fine, and if intuition directs the
healer to move other stones with it, she does so. A stone that feels
good when first placed on the body can change when its energy is
absorbed. If a stone rolls from where the healer puts it, she leaves
it where it stops, and if it rolls off completely the stone is not useful
for that healing. The two women work together in close rapport,
determining which stones are useful, and where and for how long in
that healing.

The purpose of a laying on of stones is to release etheric,
emotional, mental or spiritual blocks to well-being. In the process,
as tensions release, the woman sometimes goes through an emotional cleansing. This usually means she will cry and want to talk
about her issues, but she may express anger or resentment. She
may clench her muscles or fists; she may laugh or panic or even
temporarily feel sicker. The healer's role is to be comforting, supportive and nonjudgmental, giving the woman safety to release these
emotions and talk. Assure her that this is part of the healing, and
that the release is positive.

When the healing is over, both women know it. The woman lies
quietly and at ease, her emotional release finished. If she has
entered the meditative state or astrally left her body, she returns to
now. Gemstones, sometimes all at once, become uncomfortable or
have a 'done' feeling, and stones roll off the woman's body un-
touched. At this point, the healer removes her remaining stones,
lifting them from the woman's chakras. She clears them by smudg-

Chakra	Body	Color	Healing Issues
Root	Physical/ Etheric double	Black	Anxiety, grounding, addictions, fear, pain, colitis, diarrhea, abortion/miscarriage recovery, menopause, moving forward, karma, death, reincarnation, past lives
Belly	Emotional	Red	Uterus, menstruation, fertility, life force, red blood, circulation, warmth, constipation, AIDS, leukemia, cancer
Solar Plexus	Lower Mental	Orange/ Brown	Ovaries, spleen, sexuality, orgasm, fertility, asthma, allergies, epilepsy, arthritis, menstruation, impressions, visualization, ovarian cysts, endometriosis, coughs
Heart	Higher Mental	Yellow/ Yellow Green	Assimilation, nutrition, ideas, energy, psychic, diabetes, digestion, eating disorders, ulcers, apathy, tiredness, will power, visualization, depression, urinary
Throat	Lower Spiritual	Green/Rose	Heart disease, blood circulation, immune/thymus, love, loneliness, self image, trust, abused childhoods, giving, compassion, receiving love, imagination, infections
Third Eye/ Brow	Middle Spiritual	Blue/Aqua	Anger, communication, expression, creativity, voice, burns, sore throats, laryngitis, choking, headaches, migraines, rape and incest recovery, inflammations, swellings, ears
Crown	Higher	Indigo/White	Endocrine balancing, menstural cycles, eyes, senses, multiple sclerosis, headaches, degenerative dis-eases, white blood cells, immune system, colds, flu, sinuses, psychic development, clairvoyance, mental, pneumonia
Transpersonal Point	Spiritual	Violet	Degenerative dis-eases, vision, immunity, white blood cells, headaches, insomnia, anxiety, calming, head, brain, stress
		Clear	Connection with Goddess, all-aura healing, channeling, knowledge, unifying, clearing, vitalizing, protection

ing in incense smoke or washing them in salt water before using them again. The woman rests quietly without the stones until she is fully present, and when she rises does so slowly. She feels spacey but relieved and good, and after a healing may want to sleep. The healer places her hands to the earth to release any energies absorbed that aren't her own.

How to place the stones for a laying on of stones healing follows. The information is from personal experience, influenced strongly by Katrina Raphaell's books, *Crystal Enlightenment* and *Crystal Healing*, which were channeled material.[4] Begin by placing a blanket or rug on the floor for the woman to lie on comfortably, leaving space to move freely around her. The room should be warm; a woman lying still chills more easily than the working, moving healer does. Use a quiet room with an optional background of unobtrusive New Age music; use candlelight at night. The woman being healed should wear loose clothing, without heavy belts or excessive jewelry: some healers want jewelry removed. Skyclad is unnecessary, but comfort is important. The healer may begin by smudging herself and the woman with sage smoke; she may also end that way.

When the woman is settled, lying relaxed on her back, legs and head straight and arms at her sides, the healing begins. First place a pattern of clear quartz crystals around her, one in each hand pointing outward or beside each hand pointing toward her body. Use more quartz crystals below her feet, pointing toward her head, and above her head pointing away from her crown or toward it. Follow intuition on the directions of these crystals, or use double terminated ones. The crystals are used to draw earth energy into the woman's body from feet to head or in the opposite direction, from crown to toes. A woman who needs grounding benefits from crystals pointing toward her feet, rather than the opposite.

Then begin with colored gemstones placed on the chakras, working from the feet up. I use a velvet bag for my healing stones and pour them out on the blanket beside the woman. The stones are a mixture of forms—rough, cut, cabachons, bead necklaces, tumbled pieces and gemstone eggs. There are several stones for each chakra/color, and half a dozen or more of thin Brazilian quartz crystals three to five inches long, single terminated.

Beginning with the feet, I place a smoky quartz crystal between the woman's ankles on the floor, other pieces on her thighs of smoky quartz, black tourmaline or hematite. Directly on her root center, across the pubic bone, I gently drape a string of hematite bead-chips. For black stones, my assortment includes a black tourmaline rod, a tumbled oval of hematite, the hematite chip necklace, a piece of tumbled tourmaline quartz, and a small black agate geode with smoky quartz crystals in the center. For red root center stones, there is less choice—a ball of rough red garnet and a tumbled piece of bloodstone. More women need calming and balancing for this chakra than energizing, and many find the red stones too 'hot' for comfort.

With the stones placed on her legs and root, the belly chakra is next. The stones I use for this area are several tumbled carnelian agates and a red (brick/orange) quartz crystal. I place the carnelians across the belly in a row running from pelvic bone to pelvic bone, and the red quartz between the root and belly centers. Women with menstrual cramps, uterine or ovarian cysts, endometriosis or fertility issues often react to these stones, some liking them while others want them removed. If a woman has discomfort from these I remove them, and put in their place clear quartz crystals or complementary colored lapis lazuli or chrysocolla pieces. A tumbled tiger-eye or orange/brown agate rests nicely between the belly chakra and the solar plexus.

On the solar plexus, my stones consist of tumbled pieces of tiger-eye, citrine, rough topaz crystals and a string of malachite beads that work nicely as a bridge between the solar plexus and the heart. Again, some women like the malachite and ask for more of it (I also have an egg), while others are uncomfortable with it. Malachite is known for its ability to penetrate issues, to bring things out from within.

The heart center gets a lot of gemstones, as heart issues are usual in women's world. I place a rose quartz egg in the hollow of the woman's breastbone and drape a string of rose quartz beads across her chest and breasts. A string of green aventurine beads fits nicely between the heart and shoulders, and a piece of tumbled rhodochrosite is good between the solar plexus and the heart. A small piece of rough kunzite and a larger kunzite rod work well with the egg or on either side of it. Emotional releases may start here, the woman becoming quieter at first. Follow her moods with caring.

For the throat chakra and across the shoulders, my primary gemstone is chrysocolla, an all-healing energy I recommend to most women. The stone is an internal healer, mood raiser, throat chakra opener and creativity stimulant. Unlike Katrina Raphael, I prefer the soft form, especially from Peru, to the crystalline gem silica. When these stones are being placed, many women begin talking about their issues. I use three or four in a line from shoulder to shoulder, and often one in the hollow of the throat itself. A string of blue topaz chips is also positive for this chakra, as are pieces of celestite, blue lace agate and aquamarine. A tumbled piece of lapis lazuli, rounded and smooth, fits well at the throat and also works with the third eye. Lapis is traditionally an all-healer, and another energy that penetrates issues, sometimes not too gently. Use it with rose quartz or amethyst in the healing.

Brow chakra gemstones are a large tumbled sodalite and a flat, rough square of moonstone, enough for the small space. Many women who initially like the moonstone want it off fairly quickly. I replace it with the sodalite or lapis which can be used for both brow and throat. Some women like both moonstone and sodalite (or lapis), and one of these could rest on the bridge of her nose against her forehead. Also use azurite, gem silica, or dark blue fluorite.

There is nowhere to rest an amethyst, my violet crown chakra gemstone, on a woman's head when she's lying down, so I put it above her head on the floor. I use several pieces of amethyst, a Brazilian egg, a Mexican point and a tumbled chunk from Canada, and place them either around the woman's head or sometimes in her hands. The clear quartz crystals, already in place, are for the transpersonal point, directing the energies of all the gemstones in flow through the chakras. The list of stones I use is just one possibility. Stones in any of the chakra colors are valuable and there are dozens of choices for each color. Follow your instincts on these, without rationalizing them.

Of the gemstones available, the geode is an interesting tool. Mine is an almost-round ball of tan rock with a hollow center, the black agate core filled with smoky crystals. Geodes draw out energy and are wonderful to put over a pain area or where energy is blocked. They also work well in massage. Mine is a small, light-weight one, perhaps as large as a golf ball, used mostly at the root center because of its tan and black colors. It is useful over any chakra. None of the stones should be heavy. Once they are placed, their weight seems to disappear into the woman's aura. When removing the stones I leave them in sight for the woman to examine after the healing, and often describe what I'm using as I place each stone. The little black geode evokes lots of interest.

If a woman needs energy, I emphasize stones for each chakra using activating, primary colors, and if she needs calming, the balancing ones. For most women I use both, letting her reactions direct which stones belong and which to remove. I use several pieces each of some stones (four carnelians, three citrines, etc.), but one piece also works. I use several types of stones for each chakra (i.e., rose quartz, kunzite, pink tourmaline and rhodochrosite for the heart

Gemstones for the Chakras

Root

Black
- Smoky Quartz
- Black Tourmaline
- Tourmaline Quartz
- Black Agate
- Apache Tear/ Obsidian
- Onyx
- Jet
- Elestials

Red
- Garnet
- Ruby
- Bloodstone
- Red Jasper
- Red Jade
- Red Spinel
- Red Quartz
- Realgar

Belly
- Carnelian
- Red Coral
- Agate
- Jacinth
- Brown Jasper
- Fire Agate
- Phantom Calcite
- Fire Opal
- Red Quartz
- Wulfenite
- Salmon Jade

Solar Plexus
- Citrine
- Topaz
- Tiger-Eye
- Hawks-Eye
- Malachite
- Peridot
- Amber
- Golden Beryl
- Yellow Jade
- Chrysoberyl
- Apatite
- Yellow Calcite
- Tourmaline
- Zircon
- Fluorite
- Green Calcite
- Tourmaline
- Zircon
- Fluorite
- Sunstone

Heart

Rose
- Rose Quartz
- Kunzite
- Pink Tourmaline
- Pink Jade
- Rhodochrosite
- Rhodonite
- Dolomite
- Pink Carnelian
- Watermelon Tourmaline
- Morganite

Green
- Aventurine
- Green Jade
- Dioptase
- Emerald
- Gr Tourmaline
- Chrysoprase
- Green Quartz
- Jadeite
- Nephrite
- Gr Obsidian
- Unikite
- Dendritic Agate

Throat
- Chrysocolla
- Turquoise
- Blue Topaz
- Blue Lace Agate
- Celestite
- Aquamarine
- Amazonite
- Blue Tourmaline
- Adventurine
- Gem Silica
- Eilat Stone

Third Eye

Indigo
- Lapis Lazuli
- Sodalite
- Sapphire
- Azurite
- Dk Aquamarine
- Star Sapphire
- Blue Spinel
- Blue Zircon
- Kyanite
- Iolite
- Bl Fluorite
- Holly Blue Agate

White
- Moonstone
- Moss Agate
- White Agate
- Chalcedony
- Selenite
- Cl Fluorite
- Opal
- Aragonite
- Pearl
- Ivory
- Phantom Quartz
- Snow Quartz

Crown

Violet
- Amethyst
- Violet Tourmaline
- Garnet
- Zircon
- Fluorite
- Jade
- Sugilite
- Alexandrite

Clear
- Quartz
- Diamond
- Zircon
- Herkimer Diamond
- Rutile

center), but one type works, too, perhaps only rose quartz. Different types of stones carry different energies within the category of their color, and a range of stones utilizes a range of gemstone energies. A healing can also be done with one piece of the same type of stone on all the chakras—eight quartz crystals for clarity, fluorites for psychic opening, or pieces of lapis for clearing issues. Clear quartz crystals are good energy conductors between the chakras, whatever combination of gemstones are used. Point them all in one direction, toward the head or feet.

When the stones are all in place, have the woman rest quietly with them for as long as she wishes. If she hasn't begun to already, encourage her to talk about her healing issues. This is the time to work with anger, withheld emotions, old hurts and tragedies, unresolved resentments. Ask her why she has a particular dis-ease or healing issue, what started it, what are the emotional roots. In this relaxed, meditative healing space, the woman knows. She talks about connections she may not have consciously made before— that her migraines come from her job, her fertility issues from ambiguity about wanting children, her asthma from fear of her father. Be totally gentle, supportive and nonjudgmental with her issues and her pain. Be caring but detached and calm.

When the issues are clear—the sources and emotions of her dis-ease—explore with her ways of resolving them. These can be suggestions for relieving stress, how to find a new job, what further information she needs to define ambiguous feelings, a resolution to forgive. Invite her to visualize, creating in her mind the steps needed to clear her body of illness. For example, in infections or flu, the woman imagines white blood cells eating up the 'bugs.' In cysts or tumors, she visualizes them shrinking until gone. For resentment, ask her to send love to an image of the person who has hurt her, watching that person's image change and the hold on her dissolve. Use guided meditation to help her draw healing light through all her chakras, releasing her illness through her crown or feet with the flow of light. Form the light in the chakra color most appropriate for her needs, or use blue, gold or clear. (Some systems use gold as the crown chakra color.) This is the place in the healing where changes are made, changes to help well-being.

One healing I did was with a woman who had Epstein-Barr Syndrome, chronic mononucleosis. The day before I worked with her, I asked her to explain to me what her body needed to do to heal her of the dis-ease. She came to me with an image of the infection flowing away and leaving her. In the healing, she was quiet while I placed the stones, only commenting that the red garnet felt good.

With all of the stones in place, I asked her what she wanted moved, but all were fine. She was deeply in the meditative state and becoming emotional.

I asked her what her dis-ease felt like, if she could make a picture of it, and she described it as gooey brown tar moving sluggishly through her body. When I asked where it had come from, she started to shake and described repeated incest experiences as a child. She had never spoken of them before. I asked her if her dis-ease was anger and pain from that time, and she said it was, a feeling of pollution, along with shame and helplessness that she couldn't protect herself. A child shouldn't have to protect herself, I told her, she should be protected. The woman cried.

When she was more composed, I told her it was time to move the tar out. I gave her the image of a ball of clear light at her feet, drawn into her feet, and as she drew it through her chakras, she pushed the tar up ahead of it. Slowly she moved the tar from her feet, to her knees, vagina, belly chakra, solar plexus and heart, filling her body behind it with clear healing light. It took several tries to move the tar from her heart to her throat, and she cried and talked about her childhood. We moved the tar past her brow and out of her body through her crown center, and it poured and poured so long that I could feel and almost see it. A stream of pure clear light came behind. I guided her to continue drawing in the light for a long time, flowing it through her body, until all the tar—her dis-ease and incest trauma—were gone. When she told me the light was totally clear, we changed the color to red, then to each of the chakra colors in turn, ending with clear light again to lift her to the stars, and clear black to ground her to the earth. She chose to draw a lot of red, for a longer time. I had her surround herself with rose-colored light, for comforting and self-love, to breathe that in and through her, then to rest.

She opened her eyes with years of pain lifted. We talked of practical things as I removed the stones: continuing the clear light meditation nightly, finding an incest recovery group, getting the rest, vitamins and nutrition she needed. I suggested wearing a piece of lapis lazuli with one of rose quartz for awhile, and gave her a piece of rose quartz. As the gemstones came off, a far more animated woman asked questions about them. She felt for the first time that her dis-ease could be healed and that she could heal it. She had not before connected Epstein-Barr, her feeling of internal pollution (the tar), with her childhood trauma. We used sage smoke together to clear the room of the heavy energy, the tar she had released.

Work on the emotional sources of dis-ease was pioneered by

Louise Hay, whose book *You Can Heal Your Life*[5] looks deeply at healing issues relevant to women. Her analyses of various problems and the emotional reasons for them bring clicks of recognition, though are sometimes overly harsh and need more consciousness. Each dis-ease and its emotional source continues with an affirmation. The affirmations are important, as Louise Hay sees healing as a process of self-love and self-forgiveness. In her terms, dis-ease is a need to forgive *someone*, not condoning wrong behavior but forgiving it, and usually forgiving oneself. This is the basis of her healing methods, and she finds "that when we really love and accept and APPROVE OF OURSELVES EXACTLY AS WE ARE, then everything in life works."[6] In a laying on of stones, or any other healing, helping the woman to accept and love herself is a central part of the process.

When a woman is able to look at her healing issues and see their emotional roots, she lets go of her suffering by accepting them. In doing that, changes are made that help her return to well-being. The emphasis on source is *not* to blame a woman for her pain or to create self-blame, but to open awareness, totally without judgment. The knowledge is a way for women to understand the implications of their issues and a place to begin working on them. If a set reason for an illness doesn't fit a particular woman who suffers from it, she seeks further to find her own causes. The causes are a beginning, but only a beginning, in her healing.

From her extensive list of emotional causes of dis-ease, Hay describes aches as a longing to be held, pain as guilt, cramps as fear, and anxiety as not trusting the process of life. Arthritis is feeling unloved, cancer is resentment and deep hurt, and heart problems are longstanding lack of joy. Ulcers are fear—as are addictions, eating disorders, breathing problems, heartburn and a host of other ills. Foot, leg and hip issues are a fear of moving forward, back issues are lack of support, and stiff necks and knees are needs for greater flexibility. "Who's getting under your skin?" is the question in skin dis-eases. Headaches are feeling inadequate to a situation, and migraines, a serious issue for many women, are resistance to feeling driven and to stress.[7] In my experience, both having them and healing them, migraines are feelings of deep inadequacy coupled with intense anger.

Dis-eases of women's reproductive system are reactions to the belittlement women face in patriarchy. The male doctrine that women's bodies are unclean has been internalized by women for too long. In Louise Hay's analysis, vaginitis is unexpressed anger at a mate, the negative side of patriarchal coupledom. Uterine, ovarian

Emotional Sources of Dis-ease

AIDS	Denial of the self. Sexual guilt. Belief in not being 'good enough.'
Allergies	Who are you allergic to? Denying self-power.
Anorexia	Denying the self life. Extreme fear.
Arteriosclerosis	Resistance, tension. Narrowmindedness.
Arthritis	Feeling unloved. Criticism. Resentment.
Back Problems	Upper—Lack of emotional support Middle—Guilt. 'Get off my back.' Lower—Lack of financial support
Bladder Problems	Anxiety. Fear of letting go (of old ideas). Being 'pissed off.'
Blood Pressure	High—longstanding emotional problem. Low—lack of love as a child. Defeatism.
Breast Cysts, Soreness	Overmothering. Overprotection. Cutting off of nourishment.
Breathing Problems	Fear or refusal to take life in fully.
Cancer	Deep hurt. Longstanding resentment.
Candidiasis	Feeling scattered. Frustration, anger. Demanding, untrusting .
Colds	Confusion, disorder, small hurts.
Female Problems	Denial of the self. Rejecting femininity.
Fibroid Tumors, Cysts	Nursing a hurt from a partner. Blow to women's ego.
Headaches	Invalidating the self. Self-criticism. Fear.
Hypoglycemia	Overwhelmed by the burdens in life. What's the use?
Influenza	Response to mass negativity and beliefs.
Menopause Problems	Fear of no longer being wanted. Fear of aging. Self-rejection.
Menstrual Problems	Rejection of femininity. Guilt, fear.
Migraines	Dislike of being driven. Resisting the flow of life. Sexual fears.
Miscarriage	Fear. Fear of the future. Wrong timing.
Multiple Sclerosis	Mental hardness, iron will, inflexibility. Fear.
Skin Problems	Old buried fear. Anxiety, feels threatened. Who's under your skin?
Vaginitis	Anger at mate. Sexual guilt. Self-punishment.
Vulva	Represents women's vulnerability.

From Louise Hay, *You Can Heal Your Life*, Chapter 15. (Condensed) and fertility issues are women's thwarted creativity (in childbearing, art or self-expression). Cystitis, frequent bladder infections, come from women's being 'pissed off' at how they're treated. Premenstrual Syndrome is classic, being credited by Hay to women's rejection of femininity. But is it the *role* of femininity in a misogynist world, the trivialization of women? If cancer is deep-seated hurt and resentment, it seems telling that so many women develop uterine and breast cancer, their creativity and nurturing turned deadly. Telling too is male medicine's reaction to these women's dis-eases, to cut out thousands of women's reproductive organs each year, half or more of them healthy. Black women are victimized by this three times as often as white women.[8]

Women need to look at Louise Hay's definitions, and not only for specifically women's dis-eases, with politically conscious eyes. The patriarchal definition of women's roles and 'place' is literally making women sick. An emphasis on Goddess-within self-love is vital in using her list, and in healing these issues. Remember again that blame helps no one, and that self-blame/guilt is the source of many of the problems. Use the information for taking stock and taking responsibility, for increasing awareness and understanding. Use it with matriarchal consciousness and self-love to make positive inner changes.

In working with these issues, a full laying on of stones to resolve emotional causes requires two women. The woman being healed lies flat with the stones on her body and the healer guides her through her issues, careful to avoid judgmental statements. Simpler laying on of stones patterns work well with meditation in self-healing. Applying a line of clear crystals from the throat to the root is possible alone, as is holding a crystal in each hand and placing them or holding them over two chakras. This is especially comforting in bed at night held over the heart and solar plexus or the heart and throat. Point the crystals upward, toward the head, and use any two centers that intuitively feel right. Meditate on the feelings and emotions that come. I often use a crystal at my solar plexus and the large kunzite rod at my heart, or kunzite at the heart and clear crystal at the throat center for this. Kunzite is a very loving energy, positive for emotional stress and balance, along with the heart/crown combination of its rose and violet colors. Chrysocolla or gem silica are positive for this work, too. So is lapis lazuli. Experiment and do what feels right. Try it before sleep, during meditations, and try it using various gemstones.

Another way of doing gemstone pattern healings is in crystal patterns, which adapt to the use of colored gemstones as well. In this case, the woman makes the pattern or most of it on the floor, then lies down inside the design. The basic patterns have wide possibilities for designing to a woman's individual needs, and are positive for self-healing.

Information on crystal patterns is being channeled by several people, with connection to Atlantis.[9] Catherine Bowman's book, *Crystal Awareness*, describes these patterns, basing them on the double triangle or six-pointed star.[10] Translated to women's healing needs, the pattern evolves from the triangle, a major Goddess and women's symbol of the matriarchies. Triangles were drawn on ancient Goddess figurines, over the vulva, along with the spiral design. The symbol was women's yoni and meant creation, birth, fertility and the life force, as well as the three-form Goddess. Using the triangle in women's healing crystal patterns seems obvious and powerful.

The basic triangle pattern is of three clear quartz crystal points (experiment with clusters, too), placing them in a yoni pattern around a seated woman. Put one crystal in front of each knee and the third behind her, aligned with her spine. All three crystals point toward the woman's body. This is a pattern Bowman recommends for meditation and 'spiritual uplift'. Its reverse, with two crystals behind the woman and the third centered in front of her, is for 'physical uplift.'[11] Again the points face the woman's body. The crystals are about a foot away from the seated woman and form an equal-sided triangle. Try these also with amethyst points, both for meditation and for calming. For the physical layout, try other gemstones, perhaps paired with clear crystals, using whatever gemstone/color energy the woman needs.

When the pattern is formed, the woman sits in the center of it, using another crystal (a personal generator or pocket crystal) to draw a line between the stones, linking them and their energy. Draw the linking line clockwise, doing it three times. The action is similar to casting a circle in women's spirituality rituals and with the same intent. A protective space is created, and with it a linking and releasing of the gemstone energies. Seated within the pattern, the woman enters meditation and opens herself to the healing.

Now put both triangles together, using two patterns, the two forms interlocking. This doubles the energies in a six-sided star. In a woman lying down within this pattern, the stones are located at her knees, elbows, and one each above her head and below her feet. All the points face upward (feet to head) and the pattern requires six clear quartz crystals. Again link the energies, but do it six times with the generator, then enter the pattern. Two women can do this together or one alone. Relax inside the pattern for no longer than ten minutes, especially the first time, then break the pattern by gathering up the crystals. Rest quietly for a few minutes before moving.[12] Also try this with amethyst points, or three clear crystals and three amethysts. Try it with colored gemstones, all the same type of stone. Try it, placing a quartz crystal or a heart-healing colored gemstone in the center, with the woman holding it or resting it over her heart chakra. Rose quartz, pink tourmaline or kunzite are recommended. Try this pattern using clear crystals when also doing a full laying on of stones.

The two-triangle pattern can again be doubled, forming a twelve-sided wheel of twelve clear crystals (plus the linking generator).[13] Use this only after experience with simpler patterns, as that much crystal energy takes getting used to. The woman using it would lie down flat within the energies, once the stones are placed. The pattern puts crystals at the following points, energy directed from feet to head: a crystal each above the head and below the feet, and a crystal at each shoulder, elbow, wrist, knee and ankle. In using the generator crystal to link the energies, make a circle connecting the stones clockwise twelve times before entering the circle. Lie inside the pattern for ten to fifteen minutes and repeat the pattern again in a week's time. To turn this into a laying on of stones, add a crystal or colored gemstone over each chakra. Doing this usually requires another woman's help.

Crystal patterns can be used with laying on of stones healing work, creating the pattern around the woman experiencing the healing. Make the crystal pattern first, then add the colored gemstones to the woman's chakras. Do the rest of the healing as in other laying on of stones sessions. In this method, or in laying on of stones without the surrounding crystal pattern, combine laying on of hands/touch healing over the woman's particular pain area.

In working, for example, with a woman who had uterine fibroid tumors, I did a laying on of stones with crystal pattern around her. Once the stones were placed and the woman comfortable within the energies, I did laying on of hands over her belly/root chakra area. In addition, I surrounded the red and orange gemstones on her lower chakras with a circle of small quartz crystals, points facing her pain area. The healing was intense, the woman resting quietly after it for some time. She had been scheduled for surgery but felt well enough after the healing to postpone it. I also directed her on visualization to shrink the fibroids.

Making such complicated healing patterns requires two women, but simpler patterns with simpler laying on of stones can be adapted for use alone. Full laying on of stones healings with or without crystal patterns also lend themselves to group healing work. In this case, do the healing as a ritual, creating sacred space by casting a circle and invoking healing Goddesses. Use candles and incense, and make an altar.[14] The woman to be healed lies flat in the center of the circle, hands to her sides, as the women of her coven create the crystal pattern and place the gemstones on her chakras. Energy raised in the circle by the group of women and the stones can be directed to the woman in the center's healing.

In a Candlemas ritual I participated in, the members of the coven did laying on of stones healing work for each other, and we directed the cone of power at the end to healing all of us and the planet. In a healing ritual or individual healing, tailor each pattern and selection of gemstones to the women involved. Some women enjoy a lot of this energy and benefit from it, while others in the group like less. One woman in our Candlemas healing fell asleep and we didn't wake her; gemstones relax some women that way. (We teased her later that we'd made her pregnant in the ritual!) Each woman reacts in ways that she needs and are right for her. Plan rituals to allow for individual differences.

In any healing work, particularly in using gemstones, the factor of intuition is major, both for the woman doing the healing and the woman experiencing it. This is a factor to develop and it grows with trust and use. When the healer 'just knows' to use or not use a particular stone on a particular woman, or 'just knows' that a heart chakra gemstone belongs on the woman's throat, she follows her hunch. It may 'just happen' in a healing that she creates a fantastical spiral array of clear crystals on the woman she is working with, omitting any colored stones at all or she decides that in order to heal she must use the stones in a particular (but seemingly illogical) way.

There is no right or wrong in a healing, and the most effective healer is the one who is open to doing what feels right at the time. She may not know the reason for her choice or actions, or looking back at it afterward may discover the reason, but in following intuition she is always right. Doing this is a form of channeling, of receiving previously unknown material through the healer's meditative state. A woman working with background theory learns to use the information loosely, fitting it to each individual she heals. No two healings are alike. Entering each healing with openness and an invitation to this intuition/channeling makes the best basis for results. With the intent to do good, good comes.

Likewise, in using laying on of stones, crystal patterns, or any other form of healing, be open to what happens. Expect nothing, promise nothing, and let the energy manifest in the ways most proper for the woman being healed. Some women feel energized, others relaxed by the work. Some talk about their issues, making connections in awareness, and have emotional releases, while others don't. While 'miracle cures' are possible and do happen, more usually the healing process is speeded up and 'cures' take place naturally and logically. Women's healing is far more natural than the 'take two pills and call me in the morning' variety. Healing here is on a deep cellular level with changes not always immediately noticeable. Rather than hiding a symptom, women's healing works with real causes and works essentially on what each woman needs. In serious illness, use healing along with standard medicine.

The deepest healing results come from imperceptible subtle levels, affecting the unseen bodies through attitude/awareness changes. The woman who comes for healing because of infertility may get pregnant afterwards or decide not to have children right now, or decide to adopt. She may clear the physical issues that block her pregnancy or open up emotional ones that need further processing. The woman with a terminal dis-ease may choose to live or die, a totally personal decision, and her body reacts accordingly, not always on conscious levels. When her issues have passed the place where physical healing is possible, the healer and her gem-stones can help the woman prepare for a conscious and integrated death.

The benefits of laying on of stones in women's healing and well-being are only starting to be felt. Women as a group are ready for this method and energy, psychically sensitive and developed enough to accept and gain from it. Women are developing the methods, learning how and when to use this form of healing, learning what it does and what are the best techniques for a given result. More complicated than working with a single crystal or one or more colored gemstones, laying on of stones is an advanced method of gemstone and crystal work, and an outcome of women's growing sophistication with healing techniques.

The method is also an outgrowth of women's awareness of the dynamics of the energy bodies and the chakras, particularly with understanding of the emotional body. By delving into the emotional/feeling roots of dis-ease and using them to make positive changes, we make a great step toward taking health into our own hands and choices. Using laying on of stones to access those emotional roots, first opening the issues and then healing them, is a breakthrough in achieving women's well-being.

Laying on of stones is perhaps the oldest method of women's healing known, yet it is only being discovered today. The skills of the ancient healers from Atlantis and the matriarchies were lost for a very long time. That they are returning to women now at the same time as Goddess is returning to the earth is no coincidence. Women's responsibility is to heal ourselves, then to go on to healing others and the planet. Laying on of stones is a tool in that healing.

NOTES

1. For more information on channeling, automatic writing, and past life/reincarnation work, see Diane Stein, *Stroking the Python: Women's Psychic Lives*, (St. Paul, Llewellyn Publications, 1989).

2. Judy Chicago, *The Dinner Party: A Symbol of Our Heritage*, (New York, Doubleday, 1979) , p. 116 ff.

3. Extensive information on the aura, four bodies and the chakras is presented in Diane Stein, *The Women's Book of Healing*. Material here is a brief overview.

4. Katrina Raphaell, *Crystal Enlightenment* and *Crystal Healing*, (New York, Aurora Press, 1987 and 1985). Highly recommended.

5. Louise Hay, *You Can Heal Your Life*, (Santa Monica, CA, Hay House, 1984).

6. *Ibid.*, p. 14.

7. *Ibid.*, Chapter Fifteen.

8. Audre Lorde, "An Open Letter to Mary Daly," in Cherrie Moraga and Gloria Anzaldua, Editors, *This Bridge Called My Back: Writings by Radical Women of Color*, (Watertown, MA, Persephone Press, 1981), p. 97.

9. Frank Alper, *Exploring Atlantis*, 3 Volumes, (Phoenix, Phoenix Metaphysical Society, 1982). See also, John Rea, *Patterns of the Whole*, Vol. I, (Boulder, CO, Two Trees Publishing, 1986).

10. Catherine Bowman, *Crystal Awareness*, (St. Paul, Llewellyn Publications, 1988), p. 81 ff.

11. *Ibid.*, p. 83.

12. *Ibid.*, pp. 93–97.

13. *Ibid.*, p. 100 ff.

14. See Diane Stein, *The Women's Spirituality Book*, (St. Paul, Llewellyn Publications, 1987) for ritual structures, and *The Women's Book of Healing*, for laying on of hands.

Chapter Two

———————⊙———————

The Ancient Art of Reiki and Laying On of Hands

Reiki is a form of laying on of hands healing with origins traced to Tibet. Some form of this energy has been known in cultures worldwide, mostly spread by oral tradition, with beginnings long before the patriarchy. Tibet was the source of much of today's healing knowledge, both of touch healing and of the four bodies and the chakras. The Tibetan system of understanding the aura and energy bodies, and of using them for healing, has become universal and is a source of women's modern knowledge.

There are theories as to how this information, known also in Native America, India, Africa, Egypt and China was discovered and taught in its beginning. Survivors of Atlantis either directly or indirectly may have developed the healing method and taught it on several continents. There may have been an ancient worldwide communications network sharing the information among geographically diverse cultures, information which was lost after the patriarchal invasions or the destruction and sinking of Atlantis. Or perhaps the information was brought here by visitors or colonists from other planets. The Dogon people of Africa describe their tribal origins as being from the Dog Star, Sirius, and bringing the knowledge with them.[1] Jose Arguelles describes such origins for the South American Mayas, also.[2] The chakra and aura system of the Native American Hopi is primarily the same healing system as is found in Tibet, South America and Africa.[3] The form of touch healing known today as Reiki has been a universal healing knowledge since at least the matriarchies.

In her book *The Reiki Factor*, Barbara Ray traces Reiki healing from Tibet, and travelling from there in two migrations, to India and China.[4] From China it reached Japan, and from there was brought to the United States in 1938 by Hawayo Takata, a woman healer.

Though pre-patriarchal India claims touch healing and the aura/bodies/chakra system as its own invention, Ray says it originated in Tibet much earlier. After India adopted it, the knowledge moved by way of Egypt to Greece, Rome and the west. From China it reached the rest of Asia, particularly Japan, and from Japan was brought to North America.

Touch healing is described in the New Testament, but the process was lost from the patriarchal worldview. The doctrine was that only god or Christ could heal. In the matriarchies it was known that anyone could learn healing, but with the repression of women and women's healing, the knowledge was submerged. In the late 1800s in Tokyo, a Bible student of Dr. Mikao Usui questioned the doctrine of 'faith healing,' asking to see it before he could believe it. The student's challenge intrigued the teacher, and he quit the ministry and his university teaching post to begin a seven-year search for the healing described in the Bible.[5]

Dr. Usui's quest took him through the ancient texts of several cultures. Obtaining a Ph.D. in Chicago, he studied scripture here and Buddhism and Zen in Japan. He learned Sanskrit to read the Buddhist texts in the original, and went to India. He found the information he sought in Sanskrit, a formula in symbols of how Buddha did healing.

The historical life of Buddha, Gautama Siddhartha (about 560 BCE) parallels the life ascribed to Christ six centuries later. More interesting to note, however, are the parallels of the life of Buddha to the Bodhisattva (enlightened Being, Goddess) Kwan Yin. Historical sources place the Chinese Kwan Yin as a later figure than Buddha, but *herstorical* research shows her beginnings derived from Nu Kwa whose repairing of the world goes back to 2500 BCE in a Goddess creation story.[6] The philosophy and stories of the life of Buddha may have been a patriarchal cooptation of Kwan Yin/Nu Kwa, and the healing described would then have had origin in the matriarchies or before. Sanskrit is one of the most ancient of written languages, the closest known language to matriarchal knowledge. What Dr. Usui sought and discovered by going back to India and Sanskrit may have been information on healing from the matriarchies.

At any rate, Mikao Usui found what he sought in India, in a Sanskrit formula. Returning to Japan, still not able to apply the formula and symbols, he underwent a twenty-one day vision quest to meditate on the information. The symbols appeared to him on the last day, enveloped in light, and he left the mountain knowing how to heal. During the next seven years, he devoted himself to healing, and began to teach Reiki to others. He left his work to a student, Chujiro Hayashi, who opened a healing clinic in Tokyo after Usui's death. Hayashi was given the information, reserved only to those initiates known as Reiki Masters, to open others to the healing symbols and the transmission of Reiki healing energy.

Reiki returned to women and the west with the work of Hawayo Takata. Takata, a Japanese-American woman from Hawaii, came to Chujiro Hayashi's Reiki clinic in 1935 with cancer. Her illness healed by a series of Reiki treatments, she asked to be taught the methods. To gain acceptance, she sold all she owned to go to Japan with her two daughters. Takata learned healing at the Tokyo Reiki Center, returning to Hawaii a year later to practice it. In 1938, knowing that World War II was coming, Hayashi initiated Takata as a Master, recognized her as his successor, and died. After forty years of practicing Reiki healing, Hawayo Takata passed the Master's knowledge on to her granddaughter, Phyllis Furumoto, in 1979, before her death in 1980. Hawayo Takata and Phyllis Furumoto have brought the Usui system of Reiki healing to the west, with a deep commitment to the tradition and responsibility of healing.

Reiki means universal life force energy, derived from 'ki,' the Japanese word for this energy. Words to name this form of healing life force are known worldwide. They are ch'i or qi in China, prana in India, mana in Hawaii and orenda in Native America; every culture has its name for this vitality or life force energy. Another way of naming it is aura, the electrical force field that surrounds the physical body, as described in Chapter One. Reiki is the universal, Goddess-within energy that fuels life and comprises the four bodies of women's aura. Its use in healing is a skill going back to the matriarchies or before and is the daughter-right of every woman.

Laying on of hands is a simple way of applying life force aura energy to relieve pain and speed the healing process, to vitalize, regenerate and calm. It's a skill anyone can learn, given some simple information. Reiki differs from laying on of hands/touch healing in its use of formal physical positions for applying the energy over the chakras. The more significant way it differs is in the opening/attunement and degree process.

Reiki is taught in a series of three steps or degrees. The beginning degree, first degree, opens the woman to the ability to channel this energy freely and teaches her the healing positions. The second degree teaches Reiki as a distance healing process, revealing formula symbols to heal those not present for the treatments. The third and final degree of Reiki, restricted to very few practitioners, confers the ability to open or attune others, the information and process of the attunements themselves. The woman who completes this third degree is known as a Reiki Master. (Why not Matron, or Teacher?) This chapter combines Reiki techniques with laying on of hands for an effective healing process, but does not contain the Reiki attunements.

The degree system in Reiki, with its patriarchal hierarchy and cost, makes the knowledge exclusive and restricted. The established cost for the information and openings of a first degree Reiki healer is $150, of a second degree $500, and of a third degree or Master $10,000. Each degree's information takes an evening or so to teach. The Master, attaining the ability to open others to the Reiki energy, goes on to charge students accordingly. If Reiki is life force healing energy, which I believe it to be, it is an energy and knowledge that belongs to all. None should be excluded from receiving healing or from the ability to help others because of the requirement for money. The nature of Goddess healing is universal, which means it is everyone's. While a Reiki practitioner could be encouraged to make a living by healing or teaching, the information should be available to anyone with positive intent, not only to those who are affluent. No scholarships are offered in the International Reiki Alliance or Radiance schools of teaching, while the Traditional Reiki Masters, students of Takata and Furumoto, have some very limited sliding scale fees.

Despite the politics and ethics here, Reiki is well worth learning, both for the woman who already uses laying on of hands and for the newcomer to healing work. In my experience, the willingness and wish to heal can be enough to open the flow of energy in a woman seeking it. The pricey Reiki classes are powerful and beautiful but are unnecessary in the learning of touch healing. The first degree Reiki seminar uses meditation-type rituals to open the channel of healing energy in the student. The rituals open the chakras from the woman's crown to her heart center by a flow of light and a flow of the Reiki energy and symbols from the teacher's hands. The chakras in the palms are the means of directing this energy for healing. This energy can also be opened by using a conscious linking of self with Goddess in a women's ritual. Or it can be practiced by a woman on her own. In Reiki the opening ritual or meditation is called an attunement.

The Reiki opening rituals direct healing energy from the teacher to the student, opening the student's healing channels by transferring the energy into the student's physical body. The woman who learns and uses laying on of hands/touch healing in any form is also opening and using the Reiki healing channel. The process of laying on of hands—the opening of that channel—and the Reiki chakra healing positions are given below. Any woman can link with Goddess and her own Goddess-within to become a channel for healing energy.

Both Reiki healing and laying on of hands are ways to transmit aura energy to relieve pain, speed the physical and nonphysical healing process, and calm the emotions. They stimulate life force vitality, giving the woman receiving it a 'charge' of energy to use where she needs it for well-being. Lack of vitality (ki, ch'i, prana or mana) is the cause of dis-ease in the nonphysical body levels, just as lowered immune response is the physical reaction to these causes. Reiki or laying on of hands stimulates life force energy, allowing the nonphysical bodies to return to 'full charge' health. Since health or dis-ease first manifest on nonphysical levels, when the aura bodies are vitalized, health returns in the physical body. The woman doing the healing draws the energy from Goddess and passes it on to the woman experiencing the healing. Both women benefit, as the healer also receives that energy and vitality as it passes through her chakras and Being. The information is not exclusive to the Christian God, to the Reiki Master, or to the woman who has $150–10,000—it is there for the taking by anyone who wants to learn it.

The first degree Reiki attunement ritual opens the student's healing channels quickly and in a beautifully stylized way. The process is a remembering, as every woman has this universal life force energy within her. By using this Goddess energy to help herself or someone else, and by using its flow to develop her sensitivities and awareness, the effects of the opening attunement can happen in other ways. Power and control grow with practice and use. When this channel for healing has been opened in the Reiki rituals or developed without them, the healer learns to draw healing energy from the universe. She receives the vitality by way of her transpersonal point chakra, in through her crown and flowing through her body. The energy flow leaves through her hands, which direct the healing by their placement on the other woman's or her own pain area or chakras. The healer in this channeling of energy does not get tired or deplete herself.

To begin a teaching of this energy, it is necessary to start with laying on of hands, a skill by now familiar to many women with interest in healing work. A sketch of the basics is given here for clarity and for women who haven't done it before. Reiki is a form of laying on of hands healing. I came to the Reiki opening ritual with five years experience in laying on of hands healing and saw the attunement as another way to describe or teach that process, a faster way to develop it. I recognized the teaching technique as something familiar, though I hadn't seen it before. As the opening attunement began, I felt heat/energy from the Reiki Master's hands over my head, first opening my crown center then flowing through the upper chakras, brow, throat and heart in turn. I felt my hands, which were placed palms together in front of my heart center, stream with a flow of power that is Goddess-within, a flow I'd used in laying on of hands healings for years.

Here is how I first experienced this energy and still teach it. First rub your hands together to cause friction, then pull the palms apart and facing each other at a distance of about six inches. After a few moments, a tingling, heat, magnetic, cold or rippling sensation happens. This is woman's aura, the Reiki/laying on of hands life energy. Play with the sensation, tossing the energy like a spongy ball or pulling it like taffy between your facing palms. Keep the hands apart, not touching each other or anything else. The feeling grows and finally fades. Try it again.

In Reiki, the thumb and fingers always are held close together. Each finger is the ending of a zone or meridian, (more on this in the chapter on Chinese Healing) and contains a plus or minus electrical energy charge. The charges alternate with each finger. By holding the fingers and thumb together, the energy field is linked, as in linking the crystals of a crystal pattern. The result is stronger power, a unified Reiki, or electrical charge for healing. Hold the fingers together in this way, palms facing, and practice raising and playing with the energy. At the end of the experiment, run your hands under cool tap water or place palms to the earth to ground the collection of energies.

Now try channeling this energy, drawing it from the Goddess-universe. Imagine a flow of light starting from above your head and moving through the chakras from crown to heart to palms. The flow runs through the upper chakras, crown, brow, throat, heart, hands. Establish the image of that flow and visualize it while holding your hands palms together. Feel the energy making a triangle with a bisecting light column running through it, points at the crown and both elbows. Hold the palms together at the height of the heart center and in front of it. Feel the flowing energy entering from above the crown, moving through the chakras to the hands and making a closed circuit with the touching palms. Feel the energy, moving in a circle, leaving the body again, returning upward through the crown center. Establish this as a continuous flow. If women are working together at this or in a group, have a woman who is experienced in touch healing or Reiki place her right palm over each woman's head in turn, drawing energy from the Goddess and transmitting it to enter through the learning woman's crown.

Now move the hands apart so that they are no longer touching. Feel the energy moving between your palms, fingers held together. Reiki energy enters through the crown and flows through the healer's third eye, throat center and heart, leaving her body through her held-apart hands. Because the hands are facing and with nothing between them, the energy circuit completes. Experience the flow, make it continuous and try changing its colors. Feel it in all of the chakra colors, including black and white, then change it to clear again. Instead of grounding the energy, place your hands on the arm of the woman next to you, or on another part of your own body if working alone. Try this process in a ritual setting, with incense, candlelight and a cast circle invoking the directions and Goddess, using a meditation that asks for the openness to heal.

Now direct the healing energy toward another living thing. Two women or a group working together are ideal, but if working alone use a pet. The energy is totally positive and beneficial, it harms none and helps all. Don't be afraid to use it, to practice it or to experiment. Place your hands, held side by side or apart with palms facing, over the pain area of another woman. If the part to be healed is small, a hand or an arm for example, have her hold it between your spread hands, but not touching them. Experience the energy without touching either yourself or the other woman. Try this a few times, grounding at the end.

Again hold your hands apart, directing a flow of energy that begins above the crown and leaves through your hands, and direct this energy into the other woman's body or pain area. Feel the energy rise and grow strong, then move your hands to physically touch the other woman. Holding both hands, your fingers held together, gently on her pain area, continue channeling the healing flow of energy for as long as you feel sensations in your hands. This can be for a few seconds or as long as half an hour, depending on strength and experience, and the ability to channel the flow of energy. By now, if you have gotten the feel of this energy flow, you are a laying on of hands healer.

For a woman who does not immediately feel the flow of energy or develop sensitivity to it, it may take some time. Here are some suggestions. First, be calm and relaxed, as much in the meditative state as possible. Treat it seriously but have fun with it, there is joy in this. Also remember that you are remembering. This energy is your birthright, your daughter-right, and it belongs to you. Know that only good comes from Reiki or laying on of hands healing energy, the ability to heal yourself and others. This should not be a scary idea, the ability to heal, as nothing from even a papercut heals without the woman's own inward ability to heal it. All healing comes from within, helped by the Goddess-within energy that is available to all. By being relaxed, not trying too hard and enjoying the process, you make it easier to learn. There is no right and wrong here, no failure, and none to blame if the energy doesn't seem to happen. Stop when tired, and try it again on other occasions. Soon it happens. Also know that the healing takes place, whether the healer feels anything in her hands or not. The woman who is being healed may feel a lot of energy, while the healer feels nothing and vice versa. The quality of the sensation is different for each healing, too.

When comfortable with the flow of energy, try the Reiki positions. (See diagrams.) This is easiest to do in a group or with a partner, but the positions are also possible alone. Also try them on animals, especially a large enough dog that your hands can't cover several Reiki positions at once. Most animals enjoy this energy, though some only allow it when they actually need it. Cats in particular resent energies other than their own. Reiki benefits animals, as well as any adult or small child, and it works wonders on failing houseplants. I've even used it on my car, Shirley, when it's cold in winter and I want her to start quickly. It works.

The Reiki body positions are used in sequence, the woman being healed lying on a flat surface on her back, relaxed, hands at her sides. Both women are clothed in most cases, and the women's jewelry can remain unless in the way. I like belts, if any, removed or at least loosened and shoes off. Do the work on a surface that's comfortable for both women, as the healer holds her hands on each Reiki position for a period of about five minutes. Try to avoid sitting or kneeling in positions that make your body uncomfortable—I've cut short healings because my back hurt or feet fell asleep. Prepare to sit in a position that is comfortable for a long time and be very relaxed. The women usually remain silent during the healing, but occasionally the same type of emotional release will happen that occurs in laying on of stones. Deal with it in the same ways. (See pages 27–31.)

In the Reiki body positions, there are three positions on the head, all of them traditional. On the body, there are nine positions (one of them repeated on both sides), six of which are traditional and three optional. These twelve total placements are done with the woman lying on her back. After these are completed, the woman

Reiki Positions

HEAD: Three Positions

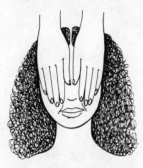

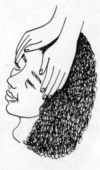

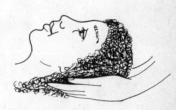

1. Third Eye -
   Across Eyes

2. Crown/Third Eye -
   Sides of Head

3. Crown - Occiput
   Back of Head

BODY: Nine Positions - Front

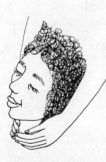

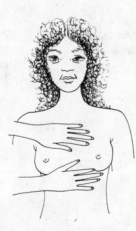

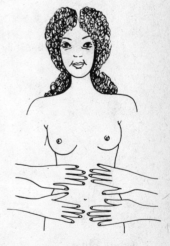

1. Throat Chakra -
   Throat, Thyroid

2. Heart Center -
   Chest, Heart,
   Lungs

3-4. Solar Plexus
   (Two Placements) -
   Lower Ribs, Liver,
   Gall Bladder, Pancreas

Reiki Positions

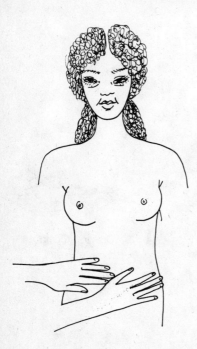

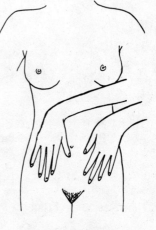

5. Solar Plexus/Belly Chakras - At waist. Stomach, Large Intestine

6. Belly Chakra - Over Pelvic Bones Uterus, Ovaries

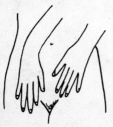

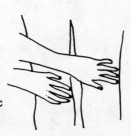

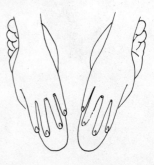

7. Root Center - Over Pubic Bone (Optional) Uterus, Vagina, Small Intestine, Colon

8. Knees (Optional)

9. Feet (Optional)

Reiki Positions

BACK : Four Positions (Plus Two Optional)

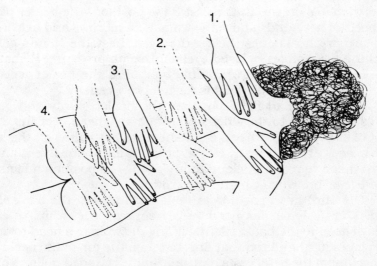

1. Heart Chakra - Over Shoulder Blades
2. Solar Plexus - Lower Ribs, Kidneys
3. Solar Plexus - Lower Ribs, Kidneys
4. Root Center - Over Coccyx

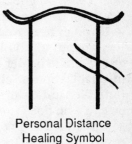

Personal Distance
Healing Symbol

turns over and there are positions done on her back. The positions closely follow the chakras and the major organ placements of Chinese healing. Exact positions can vary slightly from teacher to teacher. They also greatly resemble the polarity balancing positions that extend and embellish them.

The healer does the three head positions sitting behind the woman she is healing. The healer is seated facing the top of the other woman's crown. In the first Reiki position, the healer places the heels of her hands above the woman's eyebrows and her fingertips on her cheekbones, below the eyes. Rest the hands gently, touching the woman's closed eyelids. Use no pressure. Remain in the position for about five minutes, or until the healer feels the energy rise and change. This is for the brow center.

For the second head position, the healer slowly and gently moves her hands to the sides of the woman's head. Her fingers in front of or over the woman's ears, she rests her palms on the sides of her face. Again, remain in the position for about five minutes, both women remaining silent and relaxed. The position affects the third eye or brow chakra and the crown.

The third head position in Reiki healing is at the back of the head. The healer slides her hands from over the woman's ears/sides of head to the back, slightly lifting the woman's head to do so. She places her hands so that fingers touch the top of the neck, and the occiput of the head rests naturally in the rounded hollows of the healer's hands. Again stay in this position for about five minutes, until you feel the energy change.

Energy in using these positions rises and ebbs. When first placing hands in the positions, the energy is slight or imperceptible, but it gradually increases distinctly, resembling the energy felt when first holding hands apart to sense the aura. It can be tingly, hot, cold, magnetic, electrical, ripply. During the positions, the healer is transferring energy from the universe/Goddess. It comes in through her crown center and leaves through her hands to enter the woman she is healing. As that energy builds, the feeling can change. The healer may be aware of a speeding up of vibrations, an intensification of cold or heat, a change of temperature or sensation. Her hands may fall asleep or ache or feel electrical shock or sweat. She does not move. In a few minutes the energy diminishes to what it felt like when the hands were first placed or disappears altogether. This is the time to move on to the next position. How long the process takes varies.

There are nine Reiki body positions, again reflecting the chakras, and the healer moves to the first of these, the throat. This is done still seated behind her, hands coming across both sides of her neck so that the fingers meet in the center, over the hollow of the throat chakra. The healer's hands are held to make a tent over the center, or can touch the throat resting gently on it, or can be placed with one hand at the front and the other at the back of the neck. A woman may find the throat a sensitive position, so be aware of her comfort.

For the second body position, the heart chakra, the healer moves to sit on one side or the other of the woman she is healing. Placing her hands one beside the other on the woman's body, or end to end (fingers of one hand at the wrist of the other) she uses Reiki healing either over the chakra/breastbone or her hands placed above the breasts side by side. This is also a sensitive position, and a private one, so use discretion here. The healing corresponds to the upper chest, heart and lungs.

There are two placements used for the next position (numbered three and four in the diagrams), located at the solar plexus. The healer's hands are held side by side over first one side then the other of the woman's lower ribs. The healer is sitting to one side of the woman she is healing, and may want to change position after the last placements. These two lower rib positions cover the liver, gall bladder and pancreas. Again she holds each position for about five minutes.

The fifth body position is again for the solar plexus, moving toward the belly chakra. The healer places her hands end to end across the woman's waist, covering her stomach, kidneys and the area of the transverse large intestine.

The belly chakra is the next position, with the healer placing her hands over the pelvic bones. This area covers the uterus and ovaries, as well as the hips and pelvic area. Reiki/laying on of hands energy will not harm the fetus if the woman is pregnant. The healer's hands point downward over the pelvic bones for this placement. Hold for five minutes.

Positions seven, eight and nine are optional but very positive completions for this part of the healing. The seventh position is above the root chakra, but as this is a sensitive and private place also, use discretion. For root center imbalances and dis-eases, however, it is very positive to use. The root chakra is the vulva at the front and is usually not to be touched. On the back though, it is the tailbone and a less private area. To do this position I place my hands on the lower abdomen above the pubic mound (not on it). The other two positions are the woman's knees and feet, and the healer has to move to reach them. She does the feet sitting below the woman and facing her, so her hands touch the small chakras at the soles. If an energy blockage happens at any time in the healing, go to the woman's feet, then back to the body sequence. An energy blockage is indicated if the woman becomes very restless in the healing once the head positions are completed. Again, hold the placement for about five minutes, until the energy flow has increased, changed and ebbed.

At this point, the woman being healed turns over on her stomach, if the full Reiki healing is done. The positions on the back correspond to the heart, solar plexus and root chakras, but on the other side of the body. The chakras are not only located on the front, but are rooted in the spinal column and go through. They look like spirals or funnels, wide parts to the front and tails to the back. The four positions on the torso are done with the heel of one hand in front of the fingers of the other. The first position is over the shoulder blades, corresponding to the heart and throat chakras. The healer sits beside the woman, one hand nearer and the other hand reaching across, so the whole width of the back at shoulder level is covered by the healer's hands.

Positions two and three are like the ones over the lower ribs on the front. The healer's hands are placed side by side first on one side, then on the other of the body. The location here is the same as on the front, over the lower ribs, covering the kidneys and solar plexus. The fourth back position is over the coccyx (tailbone) with hands end to end again. This position, where the buttocks meet the back, is for the root and belly chakras. While it may be too sensitive to touch body parts on the front for the heart (between the woman's breasts) and root (her pubic bone), the positions on the back reach these centers with less sensitivity.

As in doing the front of the body, the last two positions are optional, not included in traditional Reiki but used by Radiance and Reiki Alliance. These are the knees and feet. There are small chakras at the backs of the knees and the soles of the feet—each have two small chakras. Doing the knees and feet connects the woman with earth energy, and is positive and important. Another optional and very logical Reiki position for front or back, is to place hands on both sides of any specific pain area. Again, as in all the other placements, hold for about five minutes.

At the end of a Reiki/laying on of hands session, let the woman rest for as long as she needs to and have her move slowly at first. The woman experiencing the healing feels good and her energy feels balanced and clear at the end. She has an increase in vitality and skin brightness and her breathing is calm and even. Pain is greatly reduced and the improvement can be permanent. Healing of wounds, incisions, burns or broken bones speeds up immensely. In chronic or serious illnesses, Reiki is usually performed in a repeated way, with the patients at the original Japanese healing clinics staying at the center while treatments are given several times a day. In chronic and debilitating dis-eases this form and method of healing is particularly positive. A Reiki healing has the effect of charging a battery and repetition keeps energy levels high. The number of times a day the treatments are given decreases as the woman's body resources recover and take over. Hawayo Takata was healed completely of breast cancer with repeated Reiki treatments done in residence in Japan, and her healing brought Reiki to the west. Reiki work is being done with AIDS patients to boost depleted energy.

Woman's body holds the cellular memory of good health within it, and the body does all it can to achieve that for as long as the woman lives. The programming occurs and is held at the unseen body levels, particularly in the etheric double. Reiki helps that cellular disposition for good health to manifest itself. The nonphysical bodies also carry past life memories that Reiki (or laying on of stones) helps to clear, and Reiki releases withheld emotions. The opening of emotional or karmic issues frees the body for physical good health, for the manifestation of positive cellular programming.

In acute illness or accidents, use Reiki or laying on of hands over the pain area immediately. There is no need to remove clothing, as this energy penetrates anything but lead or iron. If an area cannot be touched, do the healing by holding the hands above it. Reiki eases trauma, shock, reduces stress and pain, and keeps tissue damage to a minimum. It prevents or lessens swelling of sprains, blistering of burns and bleeding. Healing occurs more rapidly with Reiki, even when a full body Reiki treatment can't be given. As in other healing methods, it can and should be used in conjunction with standard medicine. The treatments generate the energy needed for physical healing, the life force vitality for the body to regenerate itself. Continue healing after the acute stage until the dis-ease/crisis is past.

Be aware in doing Reiki, or any other form of healing, of the nature of healing itself. No healer heals another woman, she heals herself. Healing occurs in the individual's Being, in the unseen energy bodies first, then manifests in the physical body. For healing to occur, the woman being healed must also desire it to occur, using her emotional body to transmit that energy into her etheric double and physical levels. The woman's own unseen aura bodies, her physical, emotional, mental and spiritual aspects, do the healing. What the healer does in laying on of hands, laying on of stones or Reiki is to offer the woman extra energy and vitality for her aura and body to use. The woman uses that energy as she chooses and needs it.

The choice for health or dis-ease is not always on conscious levels. If a woman consciously or not has chosen to die, no healer can prevent it. If she has chosen to live, she can heal despite great odds, as long as physical degeneration hasn't reached the no-return point. Some women, consciously or not, choose to keep a dis-ease because it brings them something else they need, like attention or caring from others. That choice may be temporary or permanent. A woman's healing issues may also be karmic ones. Some women refuse the healing energy because it too deeply threatens their system of beliefs. The healer offers her skills, channels the Reiki/Goddess-within energy, but the woman herself chooses the results.

Healers need to be aware that when they do a healing they are claiming women's power, but it is not they who cause or control what happens. The energy that the healer draws on is everyone's. She uses it, becoming a channel for transmitting the universal life force energy for someone else to use. The woman being healed heals herself, by making use of the extra vitality. Healers must be very clear about the distinctions, validating their skill but not allowing ego to interfere. A healing is a three-way partnership between the healer, the woman receiving the healing, and the Goddess/Goddess-within life force energy being tapped. Remember that it is women's daughter-right to tap that energy, that everyone can learn to heal.

Reiki is a natural for group healing work. If there are enough women doing the healing, each places her hands on one of the Reiki positions, doing the front of the body first. One woman only does all of the head placements. If there are two women working with a third, one healer starts at the woman's head while the other begins with her solar plexus. Both move down. One woman can do the placements on the head and body, while another holds the woman's feet and remains at that position. The placements are always done moving downward, in the head to feet direction.

I experienced a group Reiki healing on a workshop trip, as a remedy for exhaustion and tension. Several women did the healing for me, which we did on a woman's bed, each working with one placement. The women were a healing group that had come to my program together, and they were experienced in group work. It felt so good, I didn't want them to stop. After, they worked on me again. It helped immensely, both in giving me energy and in calming before-program stage fright.

In another Reiki healing I experienced, two friends did the healing on my floor at home. One did all of the head and upper body positions, while the other began at the waist, and moved to pelvis, knees and feet. This was a demonstration, rather than for a healing issue. As they worked, I felt a great warmth moving through me, through all of my body, not only in the places being touched. At the end of it I felt fully calm, all physical and emotional tensions lifted. The feeling of being balanced and centered lasted for several days. A full Reiki healing treats every organ of the body.

Reiki can be used in self-healing as well as in healing others. Once the energy channel has been established, the beginning healer benefits by working on herself. Do a Reiki self-healing on any pain area, anywhere you can reach. If only one hand can reach the area, do it also, placing the other hand somewhere on the body to close the energy circuit. In using one hand, this energy circuit means that most women receive energy from the left side and send it from the right. (Some women are the opposite.) When doing a self-healing with only one hand, be aware of the direction and energy of the circuit and make use of it. Healing with both hands creates the whole energy circle, rather than half of it, so place both hands somewhere on the body, even if both don't reach the pain area.

While Reiki is not traditionally done using crystals or gemstones, one-handed healings are amplified if a crystal is held in the receiving hand (usually left) and the sending (right) hand is held over the pain area. On some women, the energy circuit is switched; do the healing accordingly. There is no right or wrong, only what works. To find out which is your receiving hand, hold a crystal first in the left. It should begin tingling in a few moments. If it does, the left is receiving. If it doesn't, switch hands. If the crystal tingles in the right but not the left, the right is probably your receiving hand. Either way, be sure to keep the fingers and thumb held together in a laying on of hands self-healing and in any Reiki healing work.

Distance healing, doing healing for someone not physically present, is the second degree of Reiki training. This is a powerful way of doing healing for others, and is also very positive in most self-healing work. It reaches all parts of the body, including what hands can't reach alone. Distance healing in Reiki or other forms is basically a process of visualization, using the higher and lower mental bodies and the brow center. The healer uses the meditative state to imagine the woman to be healed standing in front of her. In simplest terms, she visualizes the woman well, mentally changing her dis-ease to well-being.

In a description of the universal process, the healer first enters the meditative state, calming her mind and her breathing. Then she imagines the woman to be healed in front of her, sometimes creating a 'viewing screen' and focusing it. When she sees the person who needs the healing, she assesses what is wrong. Asking to see pain areas or chakras, she observes the problem, what chakra is affected or where the pain area is, and the extent of the dis-ease. Then she makes mental changes in the image to correct it. If the woman has a headache and the healer sees that as a red blur around her head, the healer sends blue light to the woman's head and aura. She directs the light until the red is gone, surrounds the woman's aura with blue light, then withdraws. At the end of her healing, she grounds the energy by placing her hands to the earth to release any excess. The colors she uses are those of the chakras and aura, the same colors used in gemstone healing.

In another form of this healing, when the woman sees what needs clearing, she visualizes the effect happening. If the healing issue is a wound, she visualizes sewing it up, the bleeding stopped, and the remaining mark on the skin disappearing. I call this method tinker-woman healing. If a bone is broken, the image is of 'Goddess tape' or 'Goddess superglue' putting it back together, the break mended and gone. Visualize a tumor or cyst shrinking until it disappears. Always see the woman in good health at the end of the visualization. This is standard psychic/distance healing.

The first time I did a distance healing using Reiki was different and unexpected. I had not been taught second degree Reiki healing, but verified later that that's what I had done. In the meditative state, I visualized the woman who had asked for energy, as I usually do. This time, however, I found myself lifting my hands palms outward and volumes of strong, clear light flooding from them to the woman's image. I saw in the air between my hands, superimposed over the woman's heart chakra, a symbol that looked like a Pi character, but with two additional, diagonal lines through one leg of the figure. I knew in the healing that the symbol was Chinese and meant peace. I have never seen this figure before and could not find it in books. I believe that women can make their own healing symbols. Try traditional Goddess figures—spiral, delta, circle, star, etc. Three powerful symbols are taught in the Reiki second degree.

The woman I was healing was enveloped in this brilliant light, and the energy poured longer than in other distance healings. My friend told me after that she had felt an immediate need to sleep and had done so. The next morning she was almost well from her flu. I do many distant healings but this one was very different. I felt energized and good afterwards—I was sure that the healing had done its job. I felt the same bright glow surrounding me as surrounded the woman I worked with.

The healing symbol is an astral doorway for sending Reiki energy through space. This energy is not bounded by distance or matter, and the woman being healed can be anywhere on the planet. She receives the energy wherever she is and chooses to accept it or not, using the life force vitality for what she needs. If I have not been asked to do distance healing for someone, I go to the woman in the meditative state and ask her astrally for permission before starting. Sometimes she refuses, in which case I withdraw. In most healings, agreement to go ahead is made in person, but this is not always possible in distance work. Ethics should be clear here; to go ahead when the woman refuses is to violate her free will. With the woman's permission, however, the Reiki symbol is a doorway that opens for the healer and the woman she is healing to transmit the energy.

There are other methods of doing a specifically Reiki healing. In the meditative state, the woman uses her hands to transmit the energy, as she would if the woman were present. One way to do this is to visualize actually doing a Reiki healing on all the positions of the image of the distant woman. Hold the palms facing outward, fingers and thumb together, and imagine your hands doing each Reiki position. Surround the woman with light streaming from the healing symbol before finishing. Also surround yourself with light, and remember to ground afterward.

Another way is to visualize the woman to be healed and shrink her image down to a very small size. Hold the image of the woman in your hands and channel energy through your palms to her whole body. Continue the flow of energy for as long as it comes. With experience, a healer knows when the work is finished and when to stop. Image the healing symbol, the one I've described or one of your own, floating above your hands and surrounding them with healing Goddess energy.

All of these variations work. You can also experiment to find your own. Once the healing channel for Reiki is opened, every distance healing becomes a Reiki healing. Enter healings without preconceptions of what to do and allow the image you see and your intuition to guide the method. No two healings are alike. I've also used Reiki and other psychic methods of healing to send a blessing to someone, who responded later by telling me she knew I was doing it and that it felt good. Several women have told me that this leaves a delightful glow that can last a few days. Sending energy to someone stressed or sad can help a lot.

Use second degree Reiki in self-healing. In the meditative state, when creating the image of a woman to be healed, imagine or visualize yourself. Use that image as you would the image of another woman, and do a Reiki healing on yourself. Shrink yourself to small size and hold the image in your hands to do the healing, or visualize placing your hands on all the positions or on the pain area. Draw the healing energy from your transpersonal point and into the chakras, directing it within. Many women working alone learn healing this way as I did and perfect it on themselves before healing others. Reiki life force energy is so totally positive that only benefit comes from using it. Since healing happens in your own bodies anyway, no matter who is doing the healing, self-healing works. Most women who are healers, however, are more effective working with others than they are at healing their own issues. Sometimes it takes another woman's objectivity to help you heal yourself. In many cases, dis-ease is a karmic issue and if you heal it too quickly the learning and reason for it are lost. This is not an excuse to avoid doing self-healing; you can take initiative and learn about your Goddess-within power.

A Reiki Master (or third degree) has the ability to open others to the channeling of Reiki energy. Symbols and formulas are involved. However, any woman with the intent to heal and the willingness to practice can learn to open that channel for herself. The channel for healing is basically the kundalini, the line (physically the spinal column) that connects the chakras and transmits energy from one center to the next. The source of that channel is the Goddess universe and women's connection to Goddess-within. Reiki is a skill that every woman interested in healing should be aware of and be able to use, the ability to tap into the universal energy of the life force.

Reiki healing/laying on of hands is positive for all who come in contact with it. It relieves pain, speeds healing and calms the mind and emotions. In a Reiki healing, both the healer and the woman being healed receive this energy and are energized and empowered by it. The healer is not exhausted by doing this work, as the energy is not drawn from herself but from the universe. The woman being healed needs only to wish to be healed and have the willingness to accept and use the energy. Whether or not she believes in Goddess healing or Reiki doesn't matter, the healing still takes place. Various scientists are seeking to understand just what happens in a psychic healing, what causes the physical changes, but it doesn't really matter. What matters is that this form of healing works, and that anyone can do it to help herself or others to have a better life. Reiki enhances well-being and women's health, and that makes it an important skill in women's healing.

NOTES

1. Robert Temple, *The Sirius Mystery*, (Rochester, VT, Inner Traditions, 1987).

2. Jose Arguelles, *The Mayan Factor*, (Sante Fe, Bear and Co., 1987).

3. Frank Waters, *Book of the Hopi*, (New York, Ballantine Books, 1963), pp. 11–12.

4. Barbara Ray, *The Reiki Factor*, (St. Petersburg, FL, Radiance Associates, 1983), p. 46.

5. This story is related in Barbara Ray, *The Reiki Factor*, pp. 47–49. Also in Paul David Mitchell, *The Usui System of Natural Healing*, (Coeur d'Alene, Idaho, The Reiki Alliance, 1985), pamphlet, p. 11 ff.

6. Merlin Stone, *Ancient Mirrors of Womanhood*, (Boston, Beacon Press, 1984), pp. 27–29.

Chapter Three

———————◯———————

Polarity Balancing

Polarity balancing is a healing system much related to Reiki. It emerged from similar origins, but was developed in this country and century for modern women's use. Named by Dr. Randolph Stone (1890–1981), an osteopath, chiropractor and naturopath, polarity draws on healing theory from ancient China and India, and on touch healing methods that are universal. Women doing touch healing and body work discover polarity balancing almost instinctively, so natural and comforting are the positions and holds. Though the books on the system are written by men, polarity balancing is practiced primarily by women.

Most polarity balancing is practiced today by women who are massage therapists or chiropractors. It was intended by Stone for medical doctors, who of course rejected it. Merging easily into massage and body work, polarity balancing is done similarly to Reiki and is a beginning of such related skills as acupressure, shiatsu, reflexology and applied kinesiology. Polarity balancing is a gentle, powerful form of women's healing and is readily learned; it is done on a one-to-one basis or in groups. While some polarity positions could possibly be used in self-healing, the full polarity session cannot be done alone. Using it in conjunction with Reiki methods is positive.

Like laying on of stones and Reiki, polarity balancing is based on the structure of the aura, this time on the way energy flows through the aura and four bodies. The energy circuit made by using both hands in Reiki is the beginning of polarity work, the jumping off place between the two skills. Polarity balancing uses a series of hand positions on a woman's body that focus on this circuit, and its positions reflect both Reiki placements and the chakras and meridians. The healer's hand placements balance the energy flows in the woman she is healing. Polarity's emphasis is on the natural laws of aura energy flows and movements, and the physical placements that balance these flows. The three major principles, rephrased in women's terms are:

1. There is a life force energy within everything that lives, known as aura, soul, Goddess-within, or Being.
2. This energy has a pattern of flow through plus and minus electrical polarities. The energy in balance and flowing freely results in women's good health. Dis-ease results from blockage or imbalance of this flow.
3. Energy is transmitted through the aura body levels from spiritual, to mental, emotional and physical manifestation.[1]

These principles are basic in women's healing, going back to Tibet, India, China and the matriarchies. Where Reiki and laying on of stones focus emphasis on one and three, polarity therapy is based on the second premise, the plus and minus flow of energy.

The concept of plus and minus is a simple way of describing an energy circuit composed of opposite/attracting charges. Calling it plus and minus in no way denotes one as good and the other as bad, as both are equal and equally important and good. Think of them more in terms of the Chinese yin and yang, in their original meanings. In this thinking, there are opposites to every force and both are required for either aspect or a wholeness of both to exist. Together the polarity pairs make a balance. Such balances are seen in complementary pairs like night and day, winter and summer, spring and fall, black and white, active and receptive or morning and evening. They are not the good vs. evil values that western missionaries placed upon them when bringing the yin and yang concept from China and Asia.

By using the plus and minus (yin and yang) energy balance, women work with the life force circuit that comprises the aura. The designations plus and minus, rather than other words, are for simplicity, denoting the differences in the pull of energy or electrical charge directions. They work within the chakra and meridian systems of Chinese healing to describe a balance of energy movement that equals well-being. Good health is a free flow of this energy through the body. When the flow is blocked, dis-ease results from a state of imbalance. Polarity balancing is designed to open energy blocks and free the flow.

With this in mind, there is an energy flow body map. A woman's body is horizontally divided into three sections, each section having an overall electrical charge and containing a plus

Polarity Charges: Horizontal Zones

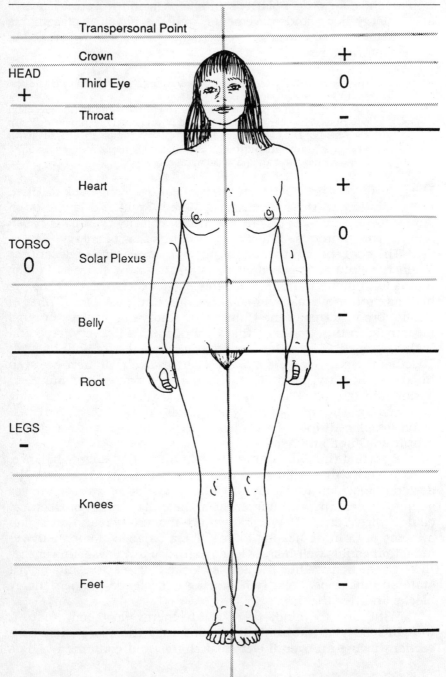

	Transpersonal Point	
HEAD	Crown	+
+	Third Eye	0
	Throat	−
	Heart	+
TORSO		0
0	Solar Plexus	
	Belly	−
	Root	+
LEGS		
−	Knees	0
	Feet	−

Polarity Charges of the Hands and Feet

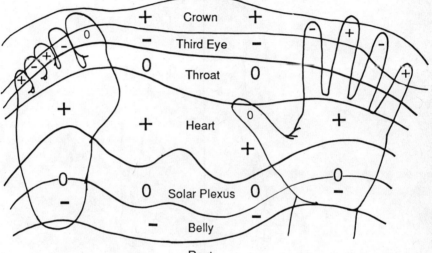

Big Toe 0	Thumb - 0
First Toe -	First Finger -
Middle Toe +	Middle Finger +
Fourth Toe -	Ring Finger -
Little Toe +	Little Finger +

Polarity Charges: Vertical Zones

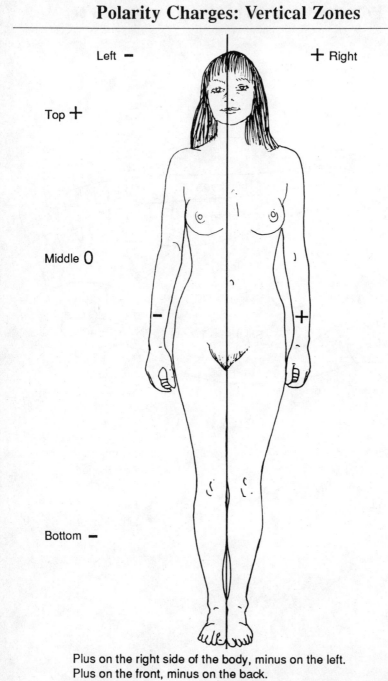

Left −   + Right

Top +

Middle 0

Bottom −

Plus on the right side of the body, minus on the left.
Plus on the front, minus on the back.
Plus on the top, neutral in the middle, minus on the bottom.

and minus energy band, divided by a band of neutral energy. The three sections are the head, body and legs, and within them and their dividing bands the energy charges alternate from chakra to chakra. If the head is the first section divided into three zones, the crown is plus, third eye is neutral, and the throat chakra has a minus charge. For the torso, the cycle repeats in the same order— plus, neutral and minus. The heart center is plus, solar plexus neutral and belly chakra minus. The bands are divided into cross-wise areas of the body, not the chakra center only. For the legs, the tops of the legs/root center is plus, from knees to ankles neutral and feet are minus.[2] Remember that there are chakras behind the knees and at the soles of the feet. The three sections each have their total charge—plus for the head, neutral for the body, and minus for the legs and feet, as well as the charges of the bands within each section.

The hands and feet are energy mirrors of the rest of the body, and sections on them also reflect the three zones, divided into horizontal bands of plus, neutral and minus charges. These are used by choosing which hand and finger to place in a polarity position on a particular part of the body. They are also used more extensively in the healing skill of reflexology, which is based primarily on the hands and feet. Each of the meridians (energy channels) of the body ends in the hands and feet, and every organ's etheric double energy is reflected in a place on them. The thing to remember for now is that the fingers and toes each have an energy charge.

Polarity therapist Maruti Seidman designates the charges of the fingers and toes as earth, air, fire, water and spirit, the points of a women's spirituality/wiccan cast circle or pentagram. In this way of describing the charges, the thumb and big toe are neutral and spirit; the first finger and toe are minus charges and air; the middle finger and toe are plus charges and fire; the ring finger and fourth toe are minus charges again and are water; and the little finger and toe are plus charges, reflecting the earth element.[3]

Running vertically, woman's energy aura body map is also divided into lines or currents, and these run in zones from head to feet. A zone ends in each finger and toe and runs in a line through the body. Healing therapies that work with these currents are sometimes called zone therapies, and include reflexology, shiatsu, acupressure, acupuncture and polarity balancing. The energy charge is plus on the right and minus on the left side of the body; plus on the front and minus on the back; plus on the top, neutral in the middle and minus at the bottom of the body. These vertical zones subdivide the energy pattern further.

With the vertical zones and horizontal body bands and sections, various points on the body also have specific charges. There are a plus and minus pair on the feet, knees, hands and shoulders, as well as breasts and pelvic bones. The energies are plus on the right and minus on the left side of the body. The chakras show alternating charges, the charges of their horizontal bands. The root is a minus charge, belly plus, solar plexus neutral, heart chakra plus, throat center minus, brow neutral, and crown chakra plus. The sections and bands of the body map reflect these individually placed charges, and the horizontal sections are more important to note in basic polarity work.

In addition to the charges, there are five major currents of energy flow: the core current, surface lateral current, diagonal current, long current and straight lines.[4] The core current flows from head to pelvis, then returns to the head in a circular pattern. Each of the currents is designated with a wiccan element, and the core current is the element of spirit or ether. The surface lateral current is a spiral covering the body from head to foot, representing air. The diagonal current runs on both sides of the body from shoulders to opposite hips, representing fire. It is part of a figure eight energy pattern. The long current splits the body in half vertically down the center, with energy swirling in opposite spirals on the two sides. This energy is the water element. The last major current is straight lines that zigzag from one side of the body to the other, vertically, with its element earth.

In polarity balancing work, the horizontal energy bands that divide the body, and the charges in the fingers and hands are the energy patterns used most. Plus sections on one part of the body harmonize with plus sections on other parts, and minus sections harmonize with other minus sections. Neutral sections are just that—neutral. When there is a block or pain area, however, the harmony is disrupted and opposite charges make an energy circuit. By placing a plus hand or finger on a minus body portion, the two hands in contact close the circuit and equalize the energy. The imbalance is relieved and the blockage opened. Placing the left hand on right body part, or minus finger on plus body part or body point, is the basis of the polarity therapy positions.

The energy theory of polarity balancing is complicated but becomes more understandable with use. Right hand to left side of the body, left hand to right side of the body is its basic application. For women like myself who have no right and left directionality ability, it begins as confusing. Yet in doing the positions, I instinctively get in flow with the energy and using the correct hand becomes

Polarity Charges within the Zones

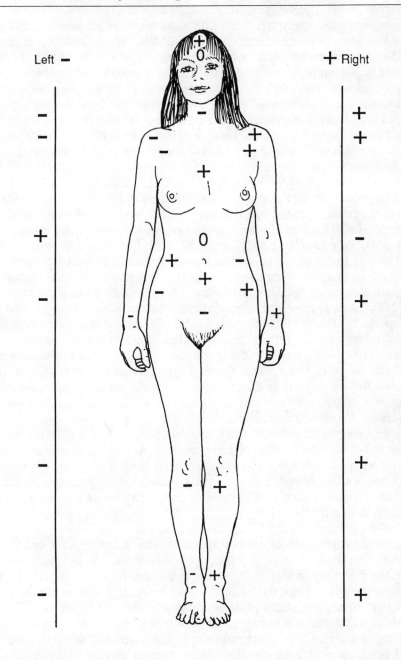

automatic—in the way that placing a hand where it hurts is automatic. Pay attention to the polarities at the start of a healing and the theory merges into practice easily. When seating myself next to a woman to begin a polarity healing, I ask her to show me which is her right hand and use that for my point of reference. In any hands-on skill, it's much more instructive to *do* a series of positions than it is to read about them, and this is particularly true in polarity work. Remember you have been doing this all along in Reiki by using two hands to complete the energy circuit. In polarity you use two hands at the same place, or one each in different places for the same result.

Polarity positions differ in a couple of ways from Reiki placements. While in Reiki, a two-handed gentle touch is used at all times, in polarity there are levels of touch. The healer can work on a particular body placement with her hands above the woman's physical body touching only her aura, with her hands touching the body as in Reiki work, or with a deeper massaging touch. Pressure is never so deep as to cause pain, as tensing the muscles is just the opposite of what polarity is designed for. Deeper touch belongs to such skills as shiatsu, acupressure, or deep muscle massage, but is not polarity. Where in Reiki the healer places her hands on a position, palms close together, and remains steady on that placement, polarity uses each hand in different positions for some of the moves, and for some of the moves there is movement or massage of the area. The combination of no touch, gentle touch and massage pressure, with palms held together or apart (but both always touching the body somewhere) differs more or less from Reiki healing positions. Polarity uses movement in some positions, stillness in others, and some of the positions are Reiki placements. It works with the chakras but the emphasis is on the energy charges. In some positions, laying on of hands/touch healing energy is used, and in others it is not. There is a combination of methods, and women also experiment.

Results in polarity balancing are very much like the results in a Reiki or laying on of stones healing. The woman who enters a polarity balancing feeling good, feels better, more relaxed, more balanced at the end of it. The more a woman needs healing, the more changes a polarity healing makes in her.[5] The technique of polarity therapy is gentle, but is slightly faster moving than a Reiki healing. Like Reiki, it regenerates and charges the life force by balancing the aura, the electrical field that surrounds woman's body and comprises her Being. The aura directs the body in creating well-being, and balancing the aura helps to release the blocks that prevent good health and cause dis-ease or illness. When the aura levels are balanced, the body falls into balance with them. The nerves relax, which in turn relaxes the muscles that they control. Relaxation of the muscles relaxes the bones, which are held by them. Bones out of adjustment can move into place in the healing. The woman is relaxed and centered, with more life force energy flowing freely through her after a polarity balancing session.

My friend Rebecca Tallman gives an example of this:

> None of the chiropractors or osteopaths in The Womb (at the Michigan Women's Music Festival) had been able to alleviate the raging headache I was experiencing as a result of my neck being out of place and pinching a nerve. In fact, despite several trips to The Womb, the pain worsened until I was nauseous, disoriented and probably a little 'shocky' from the pain.
>
> Finally a body worker offered to help, saying she not only did massage, but meridian work and polarity balancing. Even though I'm a healer myself, using primarily herbs, I had always looked askance at some of the more esoteric healing methods, but I was so miserable I was ready to try anything.
>
> Nothing has ever worked so well! (Not even pain killing drugs with codeine!) It got rid of the excruciating pain and left me feeling good—really high energy—instead of the dull, sick, wiped-out feeling I'm usually left with after the pain subsides.
>
> Needless to say—I'm a believer now!

As in Reiki, the release of energy blocks can mean the release of emotional ones. The woman experiencing a polarity balancing can have the same type of emotional release that is common in a laying on of stones or Reiki. She may cry, get angry, shake. After the healing she may want to sleep, the release completed and the emotional blocks opened. The woman in a healing may feel hot or cold, feel parts of her body tingling, or get giddy. Whatever happens is okay, and the woman doing the healing reassures and comforts her. "Life force does not differentiate between physical and emotional pain. Both are simply expressions of blocked life force."[6] A polarity balancing releases the blocks and balances aura energy, allowing the body to manifest well-being.

Polarity balancing relieves pain, calms and energizes immediately. Chronic conditions, as in Reiki healing, require repeated sessions. Use polarity in the same way as Reiki, with repeated treatments at first, lessening in frequency as the woman feels better. The longer a condition has been present, the longer it may take for results. Richard Gordon, in *Your Healing Hands* suggests:

A polarity session three or four times a week can work wonders. When the condition has shown definite signs of improvement, two polarities a week will suffice. For those who appear to be healed, one polarity a week as a tonic is an excellent idea until all symptoms are completely eliminated.[7]

Polarity balancing is recommended for all adults and children, as well as for elders. For crones I recommend that you go slow, with frequent short sessions rather than longer ones. Sustained sessions release toxins from the body, sometimes more than a woman can comfortably withstand. Do it in shorter, more frequent healings for slower, gentler results. I have also done polarity work with animals with good response.

Begin a polarity healing in a quiet room with no ringing phones or distractions. Both women are clothed, but the woman being healed takes her shoes off and should be wearing loose comfortable clothing. Richard Gordon recommends that the healer also be barefoot, for connection with the earth, and that the woman receiving the healing remove all jewelry and metal from her body and clothing. The conductive properties of metal slightly deflect aura energy. The woman experiencing the polarity balancing lies on her back, hands to her sides, and relaxes as completely and totally as possible. She can lie on a massage table, probably the most comfortable for the healer in any body touch healing, or on a bed or floor. Both women should be fully relaxed from the start. Try some deep breathing to center yourself.

The following positions for a beginning polarity balancing session are from *Your Healing Hands*.[8] Remember that the right hand touches a part of the woman's body on the left, and that placements done on one side of the body are repeated on the other. Where placements are right to right, as in the first position, harmonizing rather than balancing takes place. Finger positions are de-emphasized in this healing sequence. Hold each polarity position for as long as the energy flows, moving when the sensations stop. Parallels to Reiki are significant, and Reiki and polarity balancing are entries into each other.

The first position in a general polarity balancing is called the Cradle Hold, and it is similar to the second head position in Reiki. Sitting behind her, put your hands very gently on the sides of the woman's head, thumbs resting above her ears, index and middle fingers reaching down the occiput to the top of her neck. The placement can also be done from the front of her ears. This is for the crown and third eye chakras and is extremely soothing and comforting. Touch lightly, as in Reiki, and hold.

The second position places your left hand on the woman's forehead and your right under her head. The middle finger and thumb holds the occipital bone to pull straight back with the healer's right hand only. Pull gently and steadily and hold. The third eye is the major chakra involved.

Move from behind the woman being healed to her right side. Place your left hand on her forehead/brow chakra and your right hand over her solar plexus. Rock her body with your right hand for a few moments, then rest hands quietly, sending Reiki healing. This is called the Tummy Rock. Use steady, gentle pressure for rocking. In all three positions, hold your hands still until the energy grows, changes and fades. Then move gently to the next placement.

The first three moves were for the upper sections of the woman's body, head and torso, and the next moves are for the lower section, her feet and legs. Balancing them helps a woman to connect with Goddess Earth, calming and centering her. Complete all the moves on one leg before changing sides to do them on the other.

In leg position one, using both hands as in a laying on of hands healing, with light or no physical touch, brush off the woman's aura from top to bottom of her right leg. Shake off the energy gathered in your hands; it feels heavy and clingy. Then holding her right heel in your left hand and placing your right hand on the ball of her foot, push back on the ball of her foot, then pull forward and downward. To pull forward, the healer moves her hands to the top of the woman's foot. Do this gently and repeat it a few times.

Next, holding her right heel with your right hand, find a sore spot on the inside heel and press it steadily, not massaging it. Support the foot upright in your left hand while doing this. Supporting the heel of the same foot with your left hand, find a sore spot on the outside of her heel and press it. Using your right hand, hold the top of her foot and rotate it. Pull each toe gently, starting with the little toe, shaking her foot. (Avoid this if the woman has arthritis or a very bad back.) Use your fisted right hand to massage the sole of her right foot with your knuckles. Massage out the sore spots.

Using the heel of your left hand, push back on the ball of the woman's right foot, stretching the tendon under her big toe. Press down on the stretched tendon, working out any sore spots. There is a small round bone on the outside of the foot between heel and toes. Put thumbs under both sides of this bone, wrapping your fingers over the top of the woman's right foot. Rotate her ankle while pressing up with your thumbs. Repeat the leg and foot positions on her left foot, moving to the other side of the woman's body.

Going back to her head, tilt the woman's head to the left, placing your left hand on her brow chakra to support it. Using the middle finger of your right hand, find the right side base of the occipital bone and press. Turn her head and repeat this on the other side, hands reversed. The place is where the back of the neck meets the skull.

From her right side and arm, use your right hand to squeeze the webbing between her thumb and first finger. Find a sore spot. With your left hand, press the inside of her arm below the right elbow to find another sore spot, toward the outside of her inner arm. Alternate stimulating the web between finger and thumb and the woman's forearm near her elbow below the crease. With your right hand, pull each finger gently.

Place your right palm over the woman's solar plexus, from her right side, and your left thumb under her collarbone. Rock with both hands, moving your thumb along the entire edge of her collarbone/throat center, left and right sides. Work out sore spots, holding your hands in place for a moment at the end. Repeat the hand and arm moves on the other side.

Finishing placements use the sending of Reiki energy. Rub your palms together before each one to raise the energy if necessary. If opened to Reiki channeling or other laying on of hands energy, the flow comes without it. Richard Gordon suggests shaking off your hands between moves, releasing the static energy that collects in the healer's hands.

First, from the right, your right hand holds the woman's left foot, and your left hand holds her right hand. Hold for as long as there is an energy sensation, then shake off your hands and move to the next position.

Again on her right, put your right hand on her left hip and your left hand on her right shoulder. Rock her hips for a few moments, then stop and send healing energy. Move to the woman's left and do it again, reversing hands. Your right hand is on the woman's left shoulder, and your left hand on her right hip. The hip is the belly chakra and the shoulder is her throat center. Repeat, again sending energy after rocking; the motion opens energy blocks and feels wonderful.

From the right again, make a fist with thumbs out. Touch your right thumb to her belly chakra, below the navel. The healer's left thumb is held over the woman's third eye, not touching her forehead. These two centers are complementary and the move balances the belly chakra with the brow center. This is especially good for women with belly chakra healing issues, dis-eases of the ovaries, fertility, sexuality or menstruation. Hold the position for as long as you feel energy.

The next position, the Crown Spread, is the same as the first Reiki head placement, except that the healer's hands are placed higher so do not cover the eyes of the woman receiving the healing. Your fingers rest just above her eyebrows, for the crown and third eye centers. Try this without physically touching the woman you are working with. Hold the position for as long as there is energy sensation, and shake off after doing it.

The woman experiencing the healing turns over to lie on her stomach, and the healer places her right hand on her root chakra (coccyx, base of spine), and her left on the woman's throat center (back of the woman's neck). Rock gently for a few moments, then hold your palms on the centers for as long as the energy continues. This balancing of the root and throat is especially good for women with back problems. Try it without touch after the rocking, holding hands above the chakras rather than directly on them.

The woman lies on her back again. Balance the woman's heart with her third eye. Raise the flow of energy in your hands, and hold your right palm over her heart chakra and your left over her forehead, not touching. The heart holds emotional pain, while the astringent third eye dissolves all negativity. Using the third eye to dissolve pain can be done with any chakra or pain area. This last sequence of positions balances the woman's chakras.

Let the woman receiving the healing rest for as long as she wishes; perhaps cover her with a blanket, while you clear the energy from your hands and ground yourself. Do this by running your hands under cool tap water, or placing palms to the earth and allowing the excess energy/released negativity to leave. Women who absorb others' pain when doing healings especially need to do this but it's a good idea for everyone. Women opened to Reiki may feel less need to do this, as the energy flows through them more readily. A healer not opened to Reiki may feel fatigued at the end of a healing, while one opened to Reiki probably will not. Keep the woman being healed from getting chilled. She will be fully relaxed, possibly asleep or near it, possibly awake and energized, possibly spacey. Let her rest until she comes back to now and is ready to get up.

When the woman is ready to sit, help her and do the following final moves. Face her seated back and with your hands on her shoulders, brush across her back so your palms cross each other at the bottom of the woman's neck, moving to her shoulders. Bring your right hand down her left side, while your left brushes down her right side. Hands cross again over her waist. Stroke her back in gradually lightening strokes until you are barely using physical touch, then do it without touching. The healer shakes energy off her hands with each stroke.

For the last move, come in front of the woman and brush her aura from head to foot, right hand down her left side and left hand down her right side. Use both hands at once and do it about ten times, shaking off between strokes. Let the woman rest and run cold water on your hands or ground yourself, placing palms to Goddess Earth. Give the woman a glass of water to help continue the flushing of toxins from her body. This is useful in Reiki and laying on of stones, also. She will probably say she is thirsty.

This brief summary of a polarity balancing is the basic general healing, with dozens of variations. I highly recommend reading Richard Gordon's *Your Healing Hands* and working from it for a beginning use of polarity balancing. Once you know the principles of the energy flows, experiment with other moves, particularly placements over the chakras. One simple way of balancing the chakras with polarity work is as follows.

For this healing sequence, use the palms of both hands, the fingers held together as in Reiki. The healing runs down the center line of the body, the line of the spinal column and chakras, so no right or left side vertically is involved. Remember that the right hand is plus and the left is minus energy, and that the top of the body is plus, the center of the body is neutral, and the lower body/legs are minus energy. Use your left hand over her head, right hand over her legs, either hand or both together over her torso. Variations of the positions involve using the thumbs only, or holding a clear crystal in each hand for the balancing process. Hold your hands four to six inches over the woman's body, not touching her. Follow intuition and don't be afraid to experiment.

The first pair of chakras to balance with each other are the belly and brow centers.[9] Place your left hand over the woman's third eye and your right over her belly. Hold until the energy rises, changes and wanes. Next do the root and crown centers, right hand over the woman's root/pubic area and left over her crown/top of head. Again hold for as long as sensations continue. The third pair to balance is the solar plexus and throat. Remember that the solar plexus is neutral (some sources list it as minus) and the throat is a minus charge (though located at the top of the body, which is a plus section). Hold your left hand over the woman's throat and your right over her waist, until the energy flow ends. For the heart center, balance it with either the third eye or crown. Your left hand is over her head and your right over the woman's breastbone. Again, hold the position for as long as there is a flow of energy.

The woman receiving this healing lies comfortably on her back. The healer holds the positions, hands above and not touching the woman's physical body, for as long as she feels tingling and sensations in her hands. Then she moves gently to the next position, shaking her hands off between placements. The woman being healed rests for as long as she needs to after, and the healer grounds herself at the end, clearing her crystals if she has used them. Try this, placing one hand steadily on the solar plexus, the left hand over it while balancing the root and belly chakras, and the right hand over the solar plexus while balancing the throat, third eye and crown with your left. Try balancing the chakras using touch/Reiki, instead of holding your hands above. I have used this healing sequence many times, and women experiencing it gain a feeling of great well-being.

Try a polarity balancing that uses individual points moving vertically. Working from feet to head, the healer faces the woman's feet. Place your left hand on the woman's right side and your right hand on her left side for the following series of positions: her feet, ankles, knees, pelvic bones, hands (or elbows), and shoulders. Then use your left hand at the woman's crown and right over her solar plexus. Also try moving from head to feet, instead of feet to head, with these positions—especially if the woman needs grounding. For the final placement, instead of your right hand over her solar plexus, try both hands spread over her third eye and crown. The sequence draws energy from root to crown and is calming and vitalizing. The woman being healed feels the energy moving upward through her body. It's a good session for exhaustion or low vitality. At the conclusion of this healing, sweep your hand through the woman's aura from her head to feet, not touching her, to clear her aura of released negativity and to ground her again. The women I have tried this with have liked it.

Another chakra balancing with polarity comes from Maruti Seidman's *A Guide to Polarity Therapy*.[10] This book is more advanced than *Your Healing Hands* and designs polarity sessions for each of the major body systems and for several specific needs, such as back problems and pregnancy. Seidman uses the technique of keeping one hand stationary in this sequence, the right hand on the woman's throat chakra (back of neck), throughout most of the session. The sequence is recommended for women with stress issues, tension or headaches.

The woman being healed lies on her stomach and the healer works from her right side. The positions are lightly touching, held for as long as there are sensations in your hands. Do the sequence quietly and slowly, allowing the woman to relax and release tension and pain. Place your left hand on the back of her neck (throat chakra), while your right hand holds her coccyx (root center, tailbone), fingers pointing downward. When sensations stop, move your right hand sideways, to rest horizontally on her root center. Rock her root for about a minute. Hold still again for another minute after rocking.

Then move your right hand to her belly chakra and repeat without the rocking, holding your hands flat. Next move to her solar plexus and repeat, to her heart at the shoulder blades and repeat. Your left hand remains at the back of the woman's neck (throat chakra). When reaching her throat center in the sequence, move your right palm to the woman's throat center and your left thumb moves to her brow. Hold the position, each position, for as long as the energy flows, then move to the next one. Transfer your left thumb to the woman's crown, holding that position again for as long as the energy flow lasts, your right hand still on the back of her neck. The sequence is calming and very relaxing and centering.

Seidman uses simple polarity sequences for various body systems and dis-eases. This next one is his session for the back.[11] Try it after doing the basic polarity sequence, when the woman is fully relaxed. Follow it with a chakra balancing. The session is done with the woman lying on her stomach.

First move to her right side, placing your left hand on her throat chakra (back of neck) and your right hand cupped over her root center (coccyx). Rock her root chakra for about half a minute, then hold your hand still for about that long again. Repeat three times.

Next place your left hand on her left shoulder and your right hand on her right hip (belly chakra). Rock each placement, shoulder and hip, alternately for half a minute and hold still for half a minute. Do this three times, then use opposite hands for the woman's opposite side and repeat.

Place the thumb and first finger of your left hand on either side of the woman's highest cervical (neck) vertebra, and the thumb and first finger of your right hand in the same way over her coccyx (tailbone, lowest vertebra). Your fingers are on the muscles beside her spine, not directly on her spinal column. Rock your right hand, moving up the woman's spine vertebra by vertebra, fingers on both sides of her spine. Repeat this a second time. Your left hand on the woman's neck remains steady. The move opens energy blocks, freeing the flow of spinal (which is also kundalini) energy.

If you find a sore spot doing this, hold your fingers on it for a moment, sending healing energy. Bring your left (neck) hand down so that one hand is above and the other is below the pain area. Lift the thumb (neutral charge) of one hand and your first finger (minus energy) of the other to create a healing current of polarities. Reverse the lifted fingers and repeat five times. This releases the pain and aligns the vertebrae both at the neck and coccyx (throat and root center) levels. Now hold the sore spot with your left hand, and with the right, bend the woman's knee to lift her foot. Find the sore spot on her arch that corresponds to the pain spot on her spine. (See the chapter on Reflexology for these correspondences.) The energy block in the woman's spine will release.

Next bend her elbow, lifting her arm and hand to behind her back. This rotates and lifts her shoulder blade, the scapula. Put your upper hand under her shoulder to support and hold it, and using your other hand massage under the scapula. Move from bottom to top of the bone. Repeat on the other side. This is good for upper back and neck pain, involving the upper thoracic vertebrae. When done for my own back problems, this is the move that relieves the pain and muscle tension. Do it after the woman is fully relaxed or is as relaxed as possible. It may take several tries to relax and release this tension. Work gently.

For hip and lower back issues, as well as menstrual problems, do the next position. Slide the woman's thigh out to a forty-five degree angle from her body. Hold her ankle with your right hand and lower her foot to her buttocks. Put your left hand over her belly chakra, just below where her buttocks begin, for support. Repeat fifteen times, gently pumping her foot to her buttocks, then do the same with her other leg. The healer is doing all the lifting here, as in other movement positions. The woman being healed relaxes and lets the healer move her legs. If she is disabled in this part of her body or there is pain in her legs or lower back, ask the woman about her comfort and only do what feels good.

In the final position of this sequence, put your right hand, palm up this time, over the woman's coccyx and use your left to slowly brush down the woman's spine. Brush the energy off her body down her torso. Shake your hands after each stroke and do it until the energy feels clear, with no more static or heaviness. The blocked and negative energy released in the earlier moves is taken from the woman's aura by doing this. Have her lie quietly while she needs to, cover her with a blanket, and rinse your hands in cool water, grounding yourself from the healing. A chakra balancing is good before finishing.

The coccyx is an interesting position in polarity therapy healing. Like the third eye, it can be used to dissolve a pain spot. To do this put the middle finger of your right hand on the tip of the tailbone, and place your left hand on any sore spot of the body above the coccyx.[12] The tailbone, root chakra, is the strongest minus energy charge on the body, being the lowest point in the minus energy band of this minus section of the body. The position is recommended for back problems, childbirth labor, tension and root chakra healing issues. It can be added to the general polarity balancing session.

The third eye or brow chakra is another center that dissolves negativity. Use it by placing the index finger of the left hand on this spot and the right hand on any pain area. Opposite to the coccyx, this placement is the strongest plus polarity on the body. The solar plexus, its neutral charge at women's energy distribution center, is also used for distributing energy through the other chakras. Several of the polarity placements that use it reflect that.

I have experienced polarity sessions twice and have given them a few times. The first time I received one was at the Michigan Women's Music Festival in 1987. The day before, I'd done an all-day workshop and more than a dozen women had come to me after it for healings. I had not begun Reiki work yet, which would have left me more energized, and with a workshop a day to give for the next few days I was totally drained. My friend Judi did the healing, on a cot in the midst of a lot of activity. Her sequence included chakra balancing and connecting points with their polarizing fingers. There was little movement or massage. As the healing progressed, I became more and more relaxed and as the tension released I wanted to sleep. It was what I needed most but there wasn't time for it, so I rested for half an hour before getting up. I felt balanced, centered, calmed and greatly energized, and the feeling continued through the rest of the festival. I slept better than usual and remained steady through the rain-soaked week of the Harmonic Convergence, several workshops and many more healings.

The other polarity session I had was some months later in Atlanta. This time the healer used pressure, almost too deeply, to release pain spots and blocks. I began to shake in the healing and felt very cold but was energized and calm at the end. I knew I had done a great deal of releasing. I had thrown my back out the week before and entered the healing in a great deal of pain. Pam's healing hands released a lot of it and were a welcome relief.

I've done polarity sessions on several women, including the chakra balancing and vertical sequences given in this chapter. I've also used polarity combined with Reiki on my dogs. I adopted a Siberian Husky from the Humane Society who was badly abused and about twenty pounds underweight when I found him. Then he got sick and almost died. When I brought him home from the vet's he was very weak, and I did polarity and Reiki hand placements on him regularly for several weeks. The dog let me do it and is now healthy and doing fine. The sessions calmed his fear, and helped him adjust to a new home.

Polarity balancing is usually a one-to-one bodywork method, less effective for self-healing than other forms of women's healing work. It works well in groups and is very positive for a women's healing circle or ritual.[13] A polarity circle requires six women, working with a seventh, using both non-touch and touching without pressure or massage techniques. Receiving energy from six women is a powerful experience and is similar to a group Reiki healing. I have participated in giving these circles and received a group Reiki healing, but have not experienced a group polarity.

The healers begin a group polarity session by touching the woman being healed, each in her designated placement. After the energy grows, changes and wanes the women lift their hands and hold them above her body, until the energy flow again dissipates. The length of the contact physically and nonphysically can take as long as fifteen minutes, so the women doing the healing remember to seat themselves in comfortable positions before placing their hands. The healing can be done on the floor, but a massage table is much more comfortable for the healers. At the end of the healing, the women shake their hands off and ground, and the woman receiving the healing is allowed to rest for as long as she needs to. Cover her with a blanket. In doing the healing, the healers touch only the woman they are working with, being careful not to touch each other in the close quarters of the placements. Robert Gordon suggests that the healers chant OM while doing the first, touching part of the healing. (Women use MA).

The healers all touch the woman at the same time. Healer one sits or stands at the woman's head and does the Cradle Hold, the Reiki second head position. Her thumbs are over the woman's ears and her fingers reach down the sides of the woman's head. Barely touch her, using no pressure.

From the right, the second healer rests her left hand on the woman's third eye and her right on her solar plexus, in the center at the bottom of her rib cage. Again, use no pressure in the touch.

On the right also, the third healer places her right hand on the woman's left pelvic bone, and her left hand on the woman's right shoulder. Once all the women are in their places, she works with the next healer to rock the woman's hips gently for awhile.

The fourth healer is on the left side of the woman being healed. She places her left hand on the woman's right pelvic bone and her right hand on the woman's left shoulder. With the third healer, she rocks the woman's hips once all the healers are in their places and have begun touching. The rocking movement is rhythmic and gentle.

Healer five is on the woman's right side. Her right hand holds the woman's left foot and her left hand holds the woman's right hand.

The last healer, number six, is on the woman's left side. She holds the woman's right foot with her left hand, and the woman's left hand with her right.

The healers may want to rub their hands together before placing them on the woman's body to raise the healing energy. Also optional is the chanting, done only while the healers' hands are touching the woman. As in Reiki positions, the healers feel energy in their hands rise, change in quality, then ebb. They hold their hands on their friend's body for as long as the energy continues. With six women channeling energy in a polarity circle through the seventh woman, the process can take a long time. The woman experiencing the healing often feels heat or energy moving through her, along with a feeling of well-being.

When the flow of healing fades, the healers together raise their hands from the woman's body and hold them above her, keeping their positions. Again wait until the sensations rise, change and fade. Then the women move their hands away all at once. While the woman who has received the healing rests, the women shake off their hands, run them in cool water, or place their palms to the ground to release the excess energy. The woman who has received the healing should be given a glass of water when she is ready to sit up, and not left alone until she is back to now. She may want to sleep or feel spacey for a few minutes, taking some time to get used to the new balance of her aura bodies.

Polarity balancing is a positive women's healing technique, not as complicated to do as it is to describe. Women who use Reiki will find themselves sending Reiki energy with each polarity position. Polarity balancing is good to alleviate pain, tension, and stress or to promote general health and wellness. It is good for chronic or acute dis-eases and can be used in conjunction with other healing methods or allopathic medicine. It is helpful for any dis-ease state because polarity therapy balances the whole aura and energy bodies, releasing the blocks that cause dis-ease. Free flowing aura energy means well-being and a polarity session increases the flow of aura energy. Specific polarity sequences work more directly for individual body systems and dis-eases of those systems. A general polarity session promotes life force vitality and well-being in the whole woman. Like Reiki, polarity balancing charges the life force, 'charging a woman's batteries' so her own natural defenses can heal her.

NOTES

1. Dr. Randolph Stone, DC, DO, *Polarity Therapy*, Vol. I, (Reno, NV, CRCS Publications, 1986), Unpaged Introduction (p. 1).

2. The horizontal energy bands are from Richard Gordon, *Your Healing Hands*, (Santa Cruz, CA, Unity Press, 1978), pp. 87–88. Their connection to the chakras is my own.

3. Maruti Seidman, *A Guide to Polarity Therapy*, (N. Hollywood, CA, Newcastle Publishing Co., 1986), p. 7.

4. *Ibid.*, p. 6.

5. Richard Gordon, *Your Healing Hands*, pp. 26–29.

6. *Ibid.*, p. 26.

7. *Ibid.*, p. 28.

8. *Ibid.*, p. 38 ff.

9. Pittsburgh healer David Speer showed me the basics of this sequence. I have added to it and revised it for polarity balancing.

10. Maruti Seidman, *A Guide to Polarity Therapy*, pp. 91–93.

11. *Ibid.*, pp. 113–116.

12. Richard Gordon, *Your Healing Hands*, pp. 100–102.

13. *Ibid.*, pp. 112–117.

Chapter Four

———————————◯———————————

Chinese Healing and Acupressure

The Chinese *Nei Jing* is the oldest known written book of medicine. Dated about 300 BCE, the book contains detailed information on the complex theories of Asian healing, the techniques of acupressure and acupuncture, the meridian system, and material on herbal remedies. The author or authors are unknown. It was the first medical textbook, and is still a source of information on the ancient ways of healing that are now being revived in both east and west. The *Nei Jing* is the written source of the healing in the past, and now being incorporated with western medicine.

Chinese healing in the *Nei Jing* was a compilation of folk tradition with the learning and writings of the dynastic court physicians. Each dynasty added its own information, expanding and even contradicting the material, until the *Nei Jing*, like the Jewish Talmud, became filled with books of commentaries and interpretations. Students of traditional Chinese medicine today study the commentaries going backward in time.

> In China today, the primary textbooks used to train traditional doctors are contemporary interpretations and clarifications of Qing dynasty (1644–1911) formulas and commentaries. These books are, in turn, clarifications of Ming dynasty (1368–1644) reworkings, which are also reworkings of earlier material. This process goes all the way back to the Han dynasty (202 BCE–220 CE). Such transmission through the dynastic pathway not only preserved and encapsulated the original sources but also elucidated and reformed them.
>
> It is for this reason that the *Nei Jing*, although it is the source of the tradition, is usually one of the last texts to be studied in contemporary schools of Chinese medicine.[1]

Written in an archaic dialect, the *Nei Jing* can be read and under-stood only with much preparation. Parts of it are no longer useful, given modern medicine, but much remains valid and the *Nei Jing* or *Inner Classic of the Yellow Emperor* is still the source of Asian healing today.

As old as the *Nei Jing* is and as reverenced as it is, Asian healing predates it by centuries. Acupuncture, the science of needle insertion to relieve pain and open blocked energy flows, is 5000 years old. Acupressure, the use of finger pressure on nerve and meridian points, is the older tradition from which acupuncture grew.[2] A yet older Chinese healing method, still practiced, is herbal healing, with 500 traditional herbs going back to ancient times and almost 6000 herbs and herbal preparations used today. The oral tradition of Chinese/Asian healing is older than the written mate-rial of the ancient *Nei Jing*, how much older no one knows. Begin-ning in China, the techniques spread to the rest of the Asia and especially to Japan.

As in other cultures, archeology traces the herstory of both China and Japan back to Goddesses and probably to the matriar-chies. Merlin Stone describes habitation of China as long as 500,000 years ago, with definite artifacts pointing to a Goddess civilization that ended some time before 4000 BCE.[3] At that time, the fabled Era of Great Purity, an age when people lived in harmony with nature, the earth and the universe was ended or ending, and this golden age of the east gave way to the Great Cosmic Struggle, the ending of the Great Purity and the loss of harmony with nature. Written texts in 1000 BCE describe the Goddess Nu Kwa as creator of the earth, universe and people, and connect her name to the Era of Great Purity.

The story of Nu Kwa repairing the universe goes back to China in 2500 BCE, and Nu Kwa is the foremother of later Goddess/Bodhisattva Kwan Yin. In the story, after a period of devastating earthquakes, fires and floods, Nu Kwa helped to repair the damage and reconnect people and the earth in harmony. Such a story of devastation and earth changes seems a common memory to early civilizations worldwide and is predicted by some New Age and Native American sources to be approaching again. Nu Kwa's image as a mermaid or serpent is repeated in the Goddess stories of Kwan-non in Japan, Yemaya in West Africa, Tiamat, Nina and Atargatis in the Near and Middle East, Chalchuihtlique in South America, and in river/water Goddesses such as India's Sarasvati and Africa's Oshun. Many of these Goddesses' stories include stories of the Great Flood. Again, the similarities of Goddesses and herstory suggest a connection of cultures.

With a Goddess culture a given, and the respect for women and the life force that always goes with it, it is possible that pre-dynastic China was once a matriarchy in the Era of Great Purity. This was the case of pre-patriarchal civilizations in Europe, Asia and Africa. The fall of the matriarchies by earth changes (possibly the ones that sank Atlantis) or by conquest may in China have been the end of the Era of Great Purity and the beginning of the Great Cosmic Struggle.

A striking piece of evidence for this is a women-only language discovered in China recently.[4] The script, still passed from mother to daughter by oral tradition and kept otherwise highly secret, is believed to be more than several thousand years old. Used exclusively by women and unknown to men, it contains a syntax very different from later Chinese language and resembles characters found on carvings going back to 1600 BCE. Women who used it destroyed their writings and papers before their deaths.

When the dynasties in China began, about 221 BCE, women were excluded from the court and from education. They continued learning through oral tradition that included the transmission of the ancient women's language that a few women still know today. This herstory fits with what we know of how culture and healing were transmitted from mother to daughter and preserved after the church forced the same restrictions on women and women's education in the Dark Ages in Europe. There is a worldwide similarity in the suppression of women and also the suppression and transmission of women's healing methods. It is quite possible that the early healing information now surviving in the *Nei Jing* came from women and the very early matriarchies, that the 'folk medicine' that became the basis for Chinese and Japanese healing was indeed women's medicine.

Wherever it came from, Chinese healing theory was used with success for thousands of years before the beginnings of western medicine. The basic tenet of this theory is in the totality of Being and the harmony and balance of all component aspects within the woman. Health is harmony, and an aspect out of balance, or an energy flow blocked, is the cause of dis-ease.[5] The physical and unseen aura bodies are intrinsic to each other. Every Asian healing method is designed to rebalance, usually by means that lessen the excess and increase what is deficient in energy. Every herb in Chinese healing has its major indications, what it does in bringing energy into balance. Acupressure and acupuncture are based on channeling energy (ki) to balance in this way, as is polarity work. A major part of the art and science of Asian healing is in the healer's ability to diagnose what is deficient or in excess.

The word that means the flow of life force in China is qi or ch'i, and in Japan it is called ki. This is the same ki as in Reiki. It is the aura energy flows of polarity balancing. The ancient nature of this concept, going back to the *Nei Jing* or further, brings polarity balancing to its probable beginnings long before Dr. Stone to ancient China, Japan or possibly Tibet, and before that to somewhere unknown. Qi or ch'i or ki is "matter on the verge of becoming energy, or energy at the point of materializing."[6] Ki is the life force, the Goddess-within that all life is made of, women's aura energy or Being. In Chinese healing, Natural Ki—this life force of each woman—is composed of three types, Prenatal Ki, Grain Ki and Natural Air Ki. Prenatal Ki is present at birth, a genetic inheritance. Grain Ki comes from nutrition and Natural Air Ki from breath. In the body, Natural Ki has four major energy directions, entering and leaving, ascending and descending. In other terms this is the pathway of the chakras or the kundalini channel of the spinal column. If any of the ki directions is blocked from its normal flow, it causes a back-up or excess in one part of the body and a deficiency in another. Dis-ease is the result.

Natural Ki is divided into many other types, five of which are major divisions.[7] Organ Ki is life force energy differentiating between organs. The heart and liver are different and have different life force. Each organ has its own ki. The second type of ki is Meridian Ki, the life force as it flows through the energy channels or pathways called the meridians. Acupressure, acupuncture, reflexology, shiatsu and polarity balancing work with the meridians and Meridian Ki. The meridian system follows the lymphatic channels of the body. Nutritive Ki is the blood, which transports nutrition from digestion to every part. Protective Ki is the immune system, which protects the body from infection and contagion brought by outside influences (germs, etc.). Ancestral or Chest Ki is the harmony of the lungs and heartbeat and is connected intimately with respiration. The balance and proper flow of these types of life force energy create good health; the disharmony or imbalance of them creates dis-ease.

Chinese healing, as women's healing, is based on prevention of imbalances and on righting them before they cause serious illness. If the woman becomes ill, the effort is made to regain that balance. The doctor in China is paid when her patient is healthy; if the patient gets sick, the doctor is not paid, as she has not done a proper job. We are all our own doctors, choosing our own well-being as much as possible and paid by good health.

Every aspect of Chinese healing is to strengthen the ki, balancing the energy flows to create well-being. Though a foreign idea to the west, Asian healing is now practiced in Communist China. It has been found in countless scientific studies to be as effective as western medicine.[8] Other than for issues requiring surgery (appendicitis, broken bones, etc.), healing methods going back to the *Nei Jing* have proven themselves. They are also non-invasive and far safer than western medicine. Most traditional Chinese healing as used today is based on herbs and acupuncture, with the emphasis on healing herbs. There are no iatrogenic dis-eases (doctor caused) or side effects in Chinese healing.

Another major concept of Asian healing and the movement of ki in the body is the ancient idea of yin and yang. Only a shadow of its original meaning has come to the west. Yin and yang is a concept of balance and harmony with the universe, the balance of opposite/complementary energies.[9] Asian healing achieves its idea of harmony through balanced opposites, the balance that the matriarchal Era of Great Purity lost to the Great Cosmic (patriarchal) Struggle. Chinese methods are an attempt to regain the Great Purity, at least in the harmony of the physical body, by balance of complementary ki energies. Yin and yang are the complement and opposite of each other and everything in existence has either a yin or yang designation for its ki. They are the plus and minus of polarity work, and the balance between the opposites of yin and yang is the natural harmony of the life force. Together yin and yang are represented in the Wheel of the Year of wiccan/women's spirituality cosmology, as the turning Wheel or changing year is the harmony of life on earth.

Night and day, the waxing and ebbing of the moon and tides, the change of seasons are all examples of the balance of yin and yang. Designating yang as hot, active, firm, assertive and bright, and yin as cold, receptive, yielding, passive and dark are the basis for the mis-emphasis that limits yang to male and yin to female in the west. The concept of yin and yang is a concept of wholeness, as in the concept of w/holistic health. Each individual, male or female, grass, rabbit or mountain lion contains a balance of yin and yang energies flowing within them. Maintaining that harmonic balance is to maintain well-being.

In Chinese and Japanese healing, yin and yang extend to the organs of the body. (Organ means function rather than the western equivalent of a bodily organ.) Dissection was illegal in China at the time the *Nei Jing* was written, and the Asian conception of physiology is based on observation rather than on anatomy. The Chinese organs correspond pretty much to western designations, but there are organs in the Asian system that have no physical correspondent. There are six yang organs and five yin ones.[10] The yang organs are gall bladder, stomach, small intestine, large intestine, bladder and triple warmer (solar plexus). Their functions are digestion, the processing and absorption of food, and elimination of wastes. The yin organs are the heart, lungs, spleen, liver, kidneys, and pericardium (heart protector or circulation-sex meridian), the cavity surrounding the heart. The yin organs in the body are responsible for producing, maintaining, transforming and regulating the body's fluids—ki, blood, jing (vitality), shen (spirit), and fluids (all liquids other than blood—lymph, sweat, urine, saliva, etc.). Six additional organs are listed as 'strange' or 'curious': the brain, marrow, bone, blood vessels, uterus and gall bladder (which is also listed as yang). Dis-eases are classified as excesses or deficiencies of ki in their designated organ/s, and the way of healing is to open the blocks that cause the imbalance, harmonizing yin and yang, the organs and ki, creating good health.

Along with the very basic concepts of ki, yin and yang and the organs is the idea of the meridians and 'strange' or 'curious' flows. These are the channels that carry ki throughout the body, and they are connected to the yin and yang organs named before. There are twelve organ-connected meridians plus two central ones (that are listed as 'strange' flows), the conception (or central) and governing vessels. The other six 'strange' flows are less used. These are somewhat connected to the chakra system, are extensions of it as channels of energy movement beyond the spinal column and through the entire body. The positions used in Reiki, polarity balancing, acupressure, acupuncture, reflexology and shiatsu all work with the meridians, the pathways of ki for each of the twelve major organs.

Hiroshi Motoyama, a doctor and healer in Japan, has devised electrical ways to map the energy flows from the chakras and meridians, and finds the two systems to be coexistent with each other.[11] When a Reiki healer works with the chakras and an acupressurist or reflexologist works with the meridians, they are using energy aspects of the same electrical/aura system of women's body. The meridian channels in turn branch into the nadis, the multitudes of tiny nerve endings in the skin. Each part of the system has its place in translating ki, life force energy, into aura or life itself, women's Being or Goddess-within. The endings or seiketsu (Japanese term) of the meridians are in the hands and feet, explaining the transmission of ki that healers send from their palms and fingers in laying on of hands or Reiki, and why the skill of reflexology, which works mostly with the hands and feet, is so effective.

"The *Nei Jing* says: The meridians move the Qi and Blood, regulate Yin and Yang, moisten the tendons and bones, benefit the joints."[12] They are the warp and woof of the weaving of the aura and four bodies, a network connecting the organs and substances of the physical body. The meridians connect the interior of the body with the exterior, and working with them on the surface causes the freeing of blocked energy flows in the organs and fluids, the yin and yang of internal anatomy. In acupuncture, needles are inserted along the meridians as a means of reharmonizing imbalances. The fine needles stimulate the meridians, reducing excesses, increasing deficiencies of ki. They move stagnant energy, cool heat and warm cold, stabilize and vitalize, balance yin and yang. Classically, there are 365 acupuncture points, 150 of which are in standard usage. There are a total of over 2000 possible points that the acupuncturist or acupressurist can use.[13]

Acupressure does the same rebalancing of energy flows, ki and yin and yang as acupuncture does, but uses finger pressure on the skin instead of needles inserted into it. It is more a laywoman's technique than acupuncture, though both forms of healing have continued to be encouraged in China and Japan as techniques open to non-doctors. Acupressure works with the organ meridians and flows of ki through them to balance the body's energy by opening blocks. It is the basic skill an acupuncturist learns before using needles, and was also a typical laywoman's folk skill in pre-patriarchal Asia and since. The emphasis is on preventing blocks from becoming dis-ease issues, and on using deep finger pressure to bring about physical, emotional, mental and spiritual balance. Polarity balancing and Reiki do the same things with the energy flows but use light touch or no touch instead of pressure.

The meridians are the ki channels of the organs, and there are fourteen major meridians used in acupressure—six that connect with yin organs, six that connect with yang organs, and two 'strange flows,' one each of yin and yang. The flows or meridians can be understood by the elements of the Chinese pentacle: water, wood, fire, earth and metal (as compared to the western women's spirituality pentacle of earth, air, fire, water and spirit). Each element contains a yin and yang pair of meridians, except the fire element that contains two pairs.[14] The 'strange flows' are yin and yang, but are not given elements. They are the centers of the circle or Wheel.

The water element is the ruler of the kidney and bladder meridians. The kidney meridian (yin) stores energy reserves and the bladder meridian (yang) regulates water/fluids distribution in the

The Elements

	Water	Wood	Fire	Earth	Metal
Element	Water	Wood	Fire	Earth	Metal
Color	Blue/Black	Green	Red	Yellow	White
Sound	Groaning	Shouting	Laughing	Singing	Weeping
Odor	Putrid	Rancid	Scorched	Fragrant	Rotten
Emotion	Fear	Anger	Joy	Sympathy	Grief
Season	Winter	Spring	Summer	Late Summer	Autumn
Taste	Salty	Sour	Bitter	Sweet	Pungent
Meridians	Kidneys (yin) Bladder (yang)	Liver (yin) Gall Bladder (yang)	Heart (yin) Pericardium (yin) Small Intestine (yang) Triple Warmer (yang)	Spleen (yin) Stomach (yang)	Lung (yin) Large Intestine (yang)
Healing Issues	Hearing, sex, bones, PMS, infertility, cystitis, low back pain, salt cravings, cold hands and feet, dry hair, fear, phobias	Headaches, eyes, migraines, spine, muscle spasms, bursitis, anger, indecision, tendons	Blood circulation, protection, heart, lack of joy/sex, depression, skin changes, temperature changes, apathy, insensitivity	Menstruation, digestion, emotional, PMS, infertility, ovulation, yeast infections, stomach, ulcers, nausea, diabetes, vomiting, eating disorders, mood swings, self-pity	Acne, eczema, dry skin, hives, asthma, allergy, sinus, frontal headaches, cold, bronchitis, constipation, diarrhea, grief, delayed menses, prosperity

body. Hearing, sexuality and the bones are healing issues for these meridians, and water element imbalances also include PMS, infertility, cystitis and kidney infections, low back pain, salt cravings, cold hands and feet, dry hair, fear and phobias. The elements reflect the yin and yang Wheel of the Year, and the life force ki as body, emotions, mind and spirit.

Wood rules the gall bladder (yang) and liver (yin) meridians. The liver is a blood purifier and assimilator of food, and the gall bladder aids digestion and distributes energy. Wood imbalances that refer to these meridians include headaches and migraines, eye and vision issues, muscle spasms, spinal issues, bursitis, tendonitis, indecision, anger and rage that is chronic. Wood rules the joints, muscles, tendons and ligaments as well as the eyes, and the emotion of anger. Like the chakras, the meridians have their corresponding attributes in an emotion, sound, taste, season, odor and color, as well as in their physical body healing issues. Too much of an attribute is yang, and too little is yin. When the yin and yang, liver and gall bladder, are in balance for these meridians, the healing of their physical and emotional issues takes place.

Fire is life force creativity and the fire element has four meridians in two pairs. The heart and pericardium (or circulation-sex meridian) are yin and the small intestine and triple warmer meridians are yang. There is no western organ designation for the pericardium, which is connected to circulation and protection, or the triple warmer, which is basically the solar plexus. The triple warmer is the three vital spaces of the chest, solar plexus and abdomen. The heart meridian is the ruler of the entire meridian system and it regulates blood circulation, while the pericardium (the cavity surrounding the heart) protects the heart from damaging blows, physical or emotional. Of the yang meridians, the small intestine processes food and eliminates wastes, and the triple warmer is the energy distribution center of the body. Fire meridian imbalances include heart dis-ease, poor circulation, lack of joy, depression, lack of sexual interest, body temperature and skin changes, apathy ('losing heart'), and insensitivity to others. Remember that heart dis-eases are literally a 'broken heart' and that the heart is the central fire of women's body.

The element earth is grounding and centering, emotional and physical balance, living in the material world. Its meridians/organs include the spleen (yin) and stomach (yang), and merging with water, earth meridians are sexuality and fertility. The spleen builds blood and the stomach digests nourishment; together they rule menstruation, digestion and emotional balance. Earth element acupressure issues include PMS, infertility, irregular ovulation, yeast infections, stomach and abdominal issues, ulcers, nausea and vomiting, diabetes, eating disorders, hypoglycemia, mood swings, lack of sympathy and self-pity.

Metal rules the large intestine (yang) and lung (yin) meridians, for health issues of elimination, respiration and the skin. The large intestine moves wastes from the body, and also refers to emotional wastes; the lungs are respiration and breathing. Eastern traditions place control of breath high among values for well-being, as the speed of breathing reflects metabolism and emotions. Healing issues for these meridians include acne, eczema, dry or chapped skin, hives, asthma, allergies, frontal headaches and sinus problems, colds or bronchitis, constipation or diarrhea, delayed menses, living in the past, grief and prosperity issues.

The governing and conception (or central) vessel pair are the two major 'strange flow' or 'extra flow' meridians. They are channels that act as energy storage vessels, drawing ki from the kidney meridian for distribution. Points on these meridians are used for calming and strengthening, for increasing the results gained from stimulating the other channels. The governing vessel is yang and runs down the back of the body. The conception vessel begins in the pelvis, emerging at the perineum (between vagina and anus) and runs up the front of the body. The conception and governing vessels follow the spinal cord path of the chakras. With the exception of the governing and conception vessels, the meridians all run to a place on the foot or hand, sometimes both, and these endings or seiketsu are the basis of foot and hand reflexology.

Using these meridians for acupressure healing means applying firm finger pressure to nerve points along the meridian pathways. Jin Shin Do differs from other acupressure techniques by its use of the eight 'strange flows' with the organ meridians. Shiastsu differs in its use of whole hands, elbows and even knees to produce the pressure, along with fingers and thumbs. Examples in this chapter are given from all types of acupressure, and are identified as clearly as possible by body locations, rather than by their meridian point numbers. Body reflexology, which massages rather than presses the points, uses the meridians but identifies the pressure points as body locations exclusively. Sources for pressure points and healing sequences are identified.

Acupressure is a healing technique that is used on a one-to-one basis, and is also very applicable for self-healing. Two hands are used in Jing Shin Do and shiatsu, but only one in body reflexology. You can use a finger, thumb or whole hand to press a

The Meridians

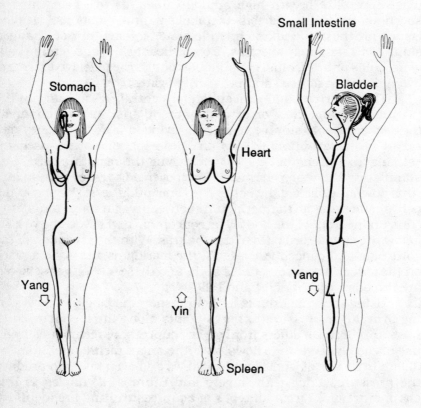

THE MERIDIAN CYCLE

The Meridians

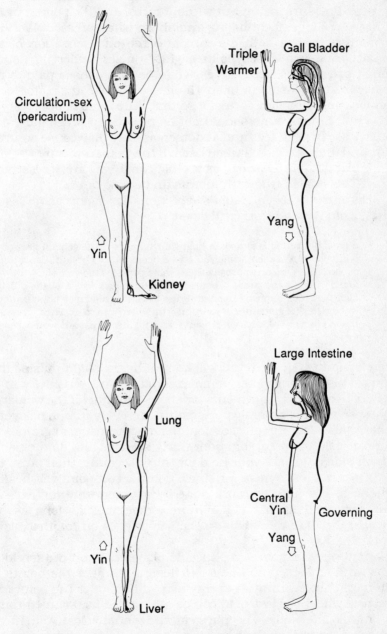

Circulation-sex
(pericardium)

Triple
Warmer

Gall Bladder

Yin

Kidney

Yang

Lung

Large Intestine

Yin

Liver

Central
Yin

Governing

Yang

point, whatever is most comfortable and provides the most even pressure. Pressure is firm but without force, and the points, which are nerve endings, feel tingling and sharp when pressed. Working the points releases both dis-ease and the odd sensation of the pressure, and a released point slightly pulses under the touch. Though pressure is used, excessive force that causes pain is not positive in acupressure or in anything else. Rather, the major focus is on locating the point correctly so that little force is necessary to unblock it. Some points should not be pressed in pregnancy, particularly on the feet, legs and abdomen as they may cause contractions, and these are noted when used. If the woman you are working with is debilitated, an elder or a child, or if you are, press more lightly. This is also true with infants and pets.

Here are Cathryn Bauer's directions for using acupressure points, from *Acupressure for Women*:

> A good beginning is simply to hold your hand over the general area of the point. Let it rest there while you take a deep, relaxed breath. Using the tip of your index finger, approach the specific point location slowly. Move your finger around the area, probing gently until you feel a slight dip that identifies the Acupressure point. Press in lightly, holding a point until you feel the tissues underneath your fingertip soften and relax. Then, press into the point very slowly, until you sense further pressure would require force.[15]

When a point is released, you will know it by the slight pulsing that begins. This pulsing takes some experience and sensitivity to be aware of. Hold most placements for about a minute. If the woman is very tense and the points very sensitive, don't try to unblock years of energy imbalance in one session. In an acute issue, migraines for example, hold the point for about thirty seconds and do the points on both sides. Release your hold for thirty seconds, then press the points again. This is more for single point or few point self-healing sequences. For full bodywork done by a woman on another, the points are held for about a minute, sometimes as long as two minutes, then are released and the healer goes on to other placements.

Acupressure points are specific placements on the meridian paths, and Chinese and Japanese healing number the points on each meridian, creating an energy map of the body. The points are on places where the flow of ki can be stimulated as it runs through the organs internally. The physical and nonphysical woman are connected, as well as the exterior with the interior of the physical. A balance of ki through the acupressure or acupuncture point results in the release of pain, dis-ease, stress and tension, an increase in vitality, immunity and calm, and an increase in general well-being. Many acupressure placements and sequences are designed for stress reduction. With practice you will learn how to find the slight depressions in the skin where the points are located, and how much pressure it takes to release them. Using the middle way (for pressure) is best. Learning touch sensitivity to find the points is half the process. In body reflexology, when you find a pain spot or sensitive area anywhere on the body, massage it out. Of course, you never use pressure over a wound or broken bone, and never use your fingernails.

A full one-to-one Jin Shin Do acupressure healing is described in Iona Marsaa Teeguarden's *Acupressure Way of Health*, and a full shiatsu healing is described in Lucinda Lidell's *Book of Massage*.[16] If you are interested in doing acupressure as a full body process, I recommend these sources. The sequences are too long to repeat here, however, and the how-to of this chapter is focused mainly on short sequences for self-healing. Be aware that acupressure is used both as a one-to-one bodywork therapy and for self-healing alone. A full acupressure bodywork session is a very positive release of pain and tension. Like a full polarity balancing or Reiki healing, it takes about an hour. Acupressure self-healing placements, by contrast, access only a few of the points of a full bodywork healing and take just a few minutes to do. Aimed at specific healing issues, they are highly effective.

The Neck Release, one of several short sequences that follows, is a placement series positive for women with headaches or migraines, as well as stress, shoulder tension or upper back pain. Compare it to polarity balancing sequences of the last chapter. Polarity placements are often the light-touch versions of acupressure ones, while acupressure placements can be more specific anatomically. The sequence is from Iona Teeguarden and is in the Japanese Jin Shin Do method of acupressure.[17] Most of the placements can be done alone.

The basic Neck Release is used to finish most Jin Shin Do full body healings. All of the points are on the woman's back and neck, and the healer uses both hands to hold both points of each pair at the same time. The first points are on the back of the shoulder blades, just below the arm-shoulder joint, in a hollow below the crest of the scapula. The second pair is in the hollows just above the shoulder blades, the tops of the scapulas. These two pairs require someone to help you, as the rest of the placements do not, and both pairs are tender spots when you locate them. The third pair is on

Acupressure

NECK RELEASE

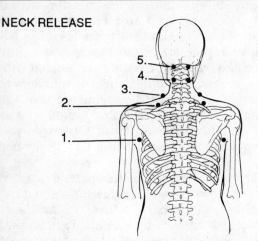

Pairs of points:

1. Below Shoulder Blades (small intestine 10)

2. Top of Scapula (triple warmer 15)

3. Neck-Shoulder Muscles (upper trapezius) (gall bladder 21)

4. Mid-Neck (non-traditional point, unnumbered)

5. Neck-Skull (gall bladder 20)

6. Web of Thumbs (non-traditional point)

7. Over Eyebrows (gall bladder 1)

8. Cheeks (gall bladder 2)

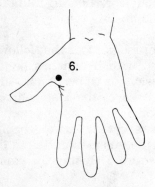

WEB OF THUMB

(Do not use during pregnancy)

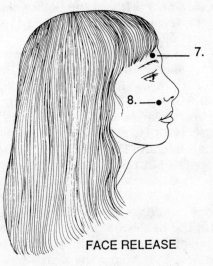

FACE RELEASE

the trapezius muscles, where the shoulders become the neck. The last two placements are on the neck itself, first on the mid-neck beside the spine between the third and fourth vertebrae. Do not press on the spinal column; the placement points are beside it about an inch away on either side. The second neck position, number five in this series, is at the base of the skull/top of neck, in the hollow between the muscles. These are two tender places against the skull. Again, the placements are beside, not on, the spine.

Hold each pair of points for about a minute, long enough to feel the energy release, a pulsing in the points. Much of women's tension is held in the neck, shoulders and upper back, and I have used this sequence at the early start of a migraine to prevent it. Other pairs of spots to use in this sequence for migraines or headaches are in the webs between the thumb and first fingers; just above the centers of the eyebrows; and at the bottoms of the cheekbones, directly below the eyes and between the nose and mouth. All of these are tender spots, in a self-healing you will know when you've found them. In a healing for others, the woman will tell you, and the healer learns to feel the dip below the skin over each placement. The sensation of putting pressure on one of these meridian points is unmistakable once you've felt it. Avoid the point in the webs of the hands if pregnant, as they may start contractions early.

Cathryn Bauer, in *Acupressure for Women*[18] gives an acupressure point sequence for menstrual pain. The first pair of points is on the back at waist level in the muscle bands beside the spinal column. The next single point is on the front of the body, directly below the navel and in line with it. Point three is on the lower legs, at the base of both calf muscles, on the inner sides of the bones (this will bring on menses, so avoid in possible/wanted pregnancy). The last pair is also on the front of the body, on the lower edges of the pelvic bones.

These four placements are the sequence, and there are additional, optional points. One of these is a single point on the back of the body, over the coccyx/root center/tailbone. Two other places are on the feet, one pair on the top center of each foot, and the other on the sides, behind the bones of the big toe. These are recommended also for indigestion. The body points are on the belly and root chakras (points one and two belly, and point five root); points three, four and seven are on the spleen meridian. The spleen or belly center is the second chakra in the chakra system.

Here is another acupressure self-healing sequence from

Acupressure

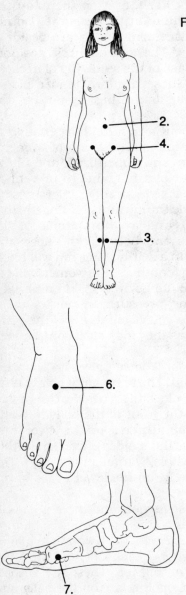

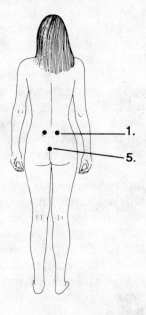

FOR MENSTRUAL PAIN AND INDIGESTION

1. Center Back (bladder 47)

2. Below Navel (conception vessel 4)

3. Lower Calf (spleen 6)
   Do Not Use During Pregnancy

4. Lower Pelvic
   (spleen 12)

5. Coccyx (governing vessel 2)

6. Top of Foot (stomach 42)

7. Side of Foot (spleen 2)

Acupressure

FOR PREMENSTRUAL EMOTIONS/PMS:

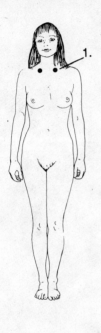

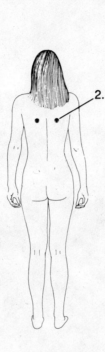

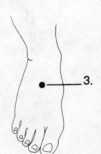

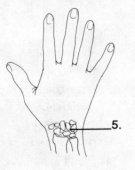

1. Under Clavicles (lung 1)
2. Under Scapula (bladder 38)
3. Top of Foot (stomach 42)
4. Side of Foot (spleen 3)
5. Wrist Joint (heart 7)

Acupressure

FOR WATER RETENTION:

FOR HOT FLASHES:

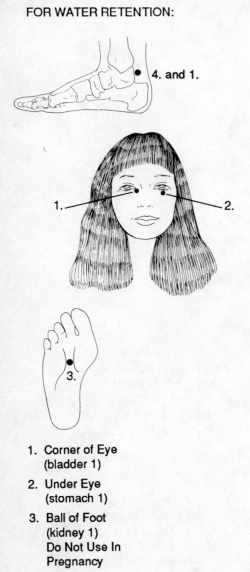

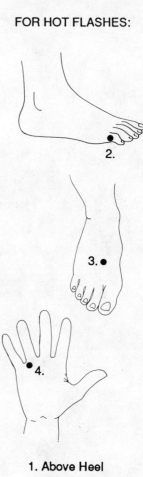

1. Corner of Eye
   (bladder 1)

2. Under Eye
   (stomach 1)

3. Ball of Foot
   (kidney 1)
   Do Not Use In
   Pregnancy

4. Above Heel
   (kidney 3)

1. Above Heel
   (kidney 3)

2. Little Toe-Side
   (bladder 66)

3. Top of Foot
   (stomach 43)

4. Ring Finger-
   Lower Joint
   (triple warmer 3)

Cathryn Bauer, this time for the emotions of premenstrual syn-drome (PMS)[19] The first point pair is under the clavicle (collarbone) where the bone meets the shoulder joints. Next is on the backs of the scapula/shoulder blades (this pair requires help to reach), on the inner edges of the scapulas. Remember rotating and massaging under the scapulas in polarity balancing. The third point pair is on the tops of the feet, the same placement as in the last sequence. Position four is behind the big toes on the sides of the feet, just behind the side of foot placement in the menstrual pain sequence. The last position is a pair on the little finger sides of the wrists, in the hollow of the wrist joints. The PMS series can be done as self-healing, except for the second placement on the back.

For premenstrual water retention, try the following self-help points, again from *Acupressure for Women*.[20] There are two point pairs on the feet and two on the face, around the eyes. The facial points occur in the inside corner of each eye, pressing sensitive spots found on the bony sockets that ring the eyes themselves. Below each eye, about three quarters of the way to the outside edge, and also on the bony sockets, find another pair of points. For foot positions, one is on the bottoms of the feet, between and almost below the round pads of the ball of the foot. The other is above the heels, on the outside of the feet next to the large tendons. The meridians these balance are stomach and bladder on the face and kidney positions on the feet. Again, avoid using foot placements if possibly pregnant, because they cause uterine contractions.

The same heel position pair is positive for relieving hot flashes, along with the following other positions. One pair is located on the side of the little toe, behind the joint. Another is just below the top of feet placements used for premenstrual emotions and pain. The last placement is on the ring fingers, outside and just below the lowest joint.[21] In reflexology, positions for every organ of the body can be found and balanced on the feet and hands. Reflexology is an-other form of acupressure.

For the woman who wants to give herself a whole body, all-chakra and all-meridian acupressure treatment quickly and with-out help, she has only to massage her ears. Meridian endings for every organ of the body are located in the outer flesh of the ears, and ear acupuncture is a science of its own in China and with acupunc-turists in the west. The ears contain a hundred acupressure/acupuncture points, obviously very close together. They are so close in fact, that best results are obtained simply by massaging the entire fleshy parts of the outside ears.[22]

The results of doing this are interesting. By using the thumb and first finger in a pinching-rolling motion to press every area of the ear flesh, you find a number of small areas that are tender or slightly painful to the touch. These are blocked meridian points, and manipulating/pressing them opens the blocks. When the process has been done, first there is a tingling warm feeling in the ears themselves, spreading to the face and then through the entire body. There is a release of tension throughout the body that almost seems impossible, considering the small portion of it you've done acupressure on. Try it and see. With so many meridians involved, only good results. The ears also have correspondences to the chakras, and acupressure/massage of them is a method of chakra stimulation and balancing.

To do ear acupressure, first hold the ear flap forward and tap behind the ear, top to bottom, with your index finger. Then,

> Starting at the tops of the ears, pinch them between the thumbs and forefingers. Doing both ears at the same time, pinch this whole area using a pinch-and-roll technique . . . You will probably find many tender reflexes as you progress along the entire ear. Tug the ears upward, keeping them close to the head. Lower your fingers to the narrow part of the ears, still using the pinch-and-roll method, and pull the ears out away from the head. Do this several times. Notice how they begin to tingle and burn.

For the lower lobes,

> Use the pinch-and-roll method of massage to pull, tug, and pinch these lobes for a few seconds . . . Then, with the fingers, start at the top of the ear and pinch and roll the outer ridge all the way around to the lobes. Now hook the little fingers in the holes of the ears and pull out in all directions. End this massage by pinching and massaging the small flap (the tragus) located in front of the ear opening.[23]

A wonderful feeling of well-being comes from doing this short process. When locating a sore spot, check the chart to see what chakra or body part is involved, and use acupressure, Reiki, polarity balancing or other forms to healing to help the flow of ki through it. Ear acupressure is probably the simplest acupressure sequence to do.

Body reflexology is based on a series of points found under the skin, usually in the areas over the organs they refer to but not always. Compare the body reflex point chart to the chart of polarity plus and minus points on the body in the last chapter. The pressure points run in a main line along the spinal column/chakra kundalini column, and points match each of the chakra centers. This center line is the conception or central vessel meridian up the front and the

Ear Acupressure

THE EAR

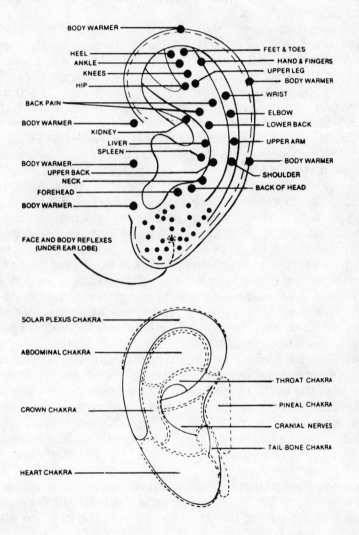

BODY WARMER

HEEL
ANKLE
KNEES
HIP

BACK PAIN

BODY WARMER

KIDNEY
LIVER
SPLEEN

BODY WARMER
UPPER BACK
NECK
FOREHEAD

BODY WARMER

FEET & TOES
HAND & FINGERS
UPPER LEG
BODY WARMER

WRIST

ELBOW
LOWER BACK

UPPER ARM

BODY WARMER

SHOULDER

BACK OF HEAD

FACE AND BODY REFLEXES
(UNDER EAR LOBE)

SOLAR PLEXUS CHAKRA

ABDOMINAL CHAKRA

THROAT CHAKRA

PINEAL CHAKRA

CROWN CHAKRA

CRANIAL NERVES

TAIL-BONE CHAKRA

HEART CHAKRA

From Mildred Carter, *Body Reflexology*, (W. Nyack, NY, Parker Publishing Co., 1983), p. 46, reprinted with permission.

governing vessel down the back of the body. The line of points running along the right side of the body follows probably the stomach meridian, and the line of pressure placements down the left side are the spleen and liver meridians. In polarity, these would be vertical energy flows.

To use these meridian acupressure points for self-healing, press in along them until you feel their locations under the skin. Some are deeper than others and it may take some searching around to find them. Use finger pressure to go beneath the fat layer, as many of the points are against bones or muscles. When finding any pressure point that is painful to touch, use your index or middle finger to hold the point or massage it for several seconds until the tenderness releases. By releasing pain in the meridian point this way, you are also releasing ki blockage or congestion in the organ it refers to. It is not the organ itself, but the meridian or ki pathway that the healing effects. If a point is very painful, hold it for a few seconds, release it for a few seconds, then hold it again. Do this no more than three or four times, then try another day.

Reflexologist Mildred Carter suggests that any pressure point that pulses when first touched (before pressure) is congested and needs finger pressure to unblock it. This is a different pulse feeling than once a point has been released, a feeling that comes only after acupressure to the meridian point. She suggests lying on your back before getting up each morning and checking the points on the abdomen and chest, releasing with pressure any painful areas, for energy and well-being throughout the day.[24] Try the placements given on the chart for a chakra balancing sequence. A point on the center of the forehead reflexes the third eye, and one just above it is a meridian line to the crown chakra. The other placements are on the body reflexology chart, and are familiar to women who have read this book so far.

For a couple of specific dis-ease suggestions, for asthma pull down while pressing inward on a point at the throat chakra, where the collarbone dips to make a V in the center of the lower throat. This helps to stop an asthma attack. Other asthma reflexes are about two inches below the collarbone V; at the third eye on the forehead; and a pair of points at the edge of the hairline where it meets the ears on both sides.[25] Note that the first three of these meridian placements are on the center line of the body, the first two on the conception vessel, and the third eye point is on the governing vessel that begins on the center line at the upper lip and goes over the head to continue down the back of the body. The pair at the ears appear to be spleen and gall bladder meridians, corresponding

Body Reflexology Points

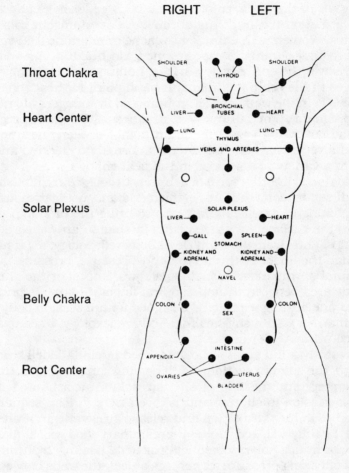

RIGHT   LEFT

Throat Chakra

Heart Center

Solar Plexus

Belly Chakra

Root Center

SHOULDER   THYROID   SHOULDER
BRONCHIAL TUBES
LIVER   HEART
LUNG   THYMUS   LUNG
VEINS AND ARTERIES
SOLAR PLEXUS
LIVER   HEART
GALL   SPLEEN
STOMACH
KIDNEY AND ADRENAL   KIDNEY AND ADRENAL
NAVEL
COLON   SEX   COLON
INTESTINE
APPENDIX
OVARIES   UTERUS
BLADDER

From Mildred Carter, *Body Reflexology*, (W. Nyack, NY, Parker Publishing Co., 1983), p. 38, reprinted with permission.

organs with the belly chakra.

For headaches, do the Neck Release acupressure sequence given earlier. If the issue is frequent headaches or migraines, try working all of the body points in the body reflexology chart. Pay special attention to the points of the kidneys, stomach, colon and intestines. Women with chronic headache or migraine issues make sure of regular elimination to prevent toxin buildup. Also do acupressure over the entire head surface, finding and releasing any ki blockages in the scalp meridians. A hand point for headaches and migraines is in the web between thumb and first fingers (do not use when pregnant). For faintness or dizziness, (OK when pregnant) press the governing vessel meridian point between the upper lip and the nose.[26] I have included more information on hand and foot points in a variety of dis-eases in the next chapter.

Shiatsu is another form of acupressure, like Jin Shin Do from Japan. It works along the lines of the meridians, using pressure and the stretching of muscles and limbs to bring the meridian points closer to the surface. Pressure points in shiatsu are called tsubos. Differing slightly from Jin Shin Do or body reflexology, shiatsu uses more than the finger or thumb to apply pressure. Pressure is done with thumbs, whole hands/palms, elbows, knees, or the grasping of a body area between thumb and first finger. Shiatsu is primarily a one-to-one healing technique, designed for full session bodywork, rather than for use in self-healing. Body reflexology, in contrast, is designed primarily for self-use.

To study a full shiatsu healing, read Lucinda Lidell's *Book of Massage*, the shiatsu section. A full healing cannot be described in this chapter, but the use of shiatsu points incorporated into a massage session is shorter and is given here.[27] The sequence is designed to induce relaxation and release stress. Begin it after the woman is fully relaxed from a preliminary bodywork massage session, or from a polarity balancing or Reiki healing. If she is pregnant, avoid using pressure on her legs or feet, the webs between her thumbs and first fingers, and on her abdomen.

Starting on the back of the woman's body, the healer begins with three pressure point pairs on the top of the back, along the shoulder blades. These are on both sides of the spinal column, not on the spine itself. Find the hollows and press the points in pairs. Compare the placements to the Neck Release. These tsubos or meridian points balance all internal functions. Two more pairs are located at the waist, again on both sides of the spinal column. One of these was used in the menstrual pain sequence. Squeeze the sides of the buttocks with both hands to relax the pelvis and open

Shiatsu Massage Sequence

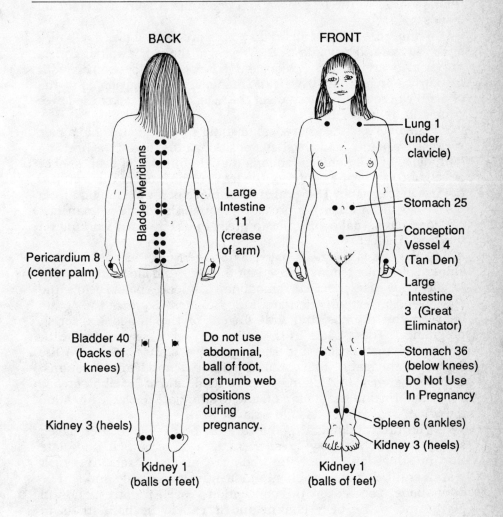

BACK

FRONT

Bladder Meridians

Pericardium 8 (center palm)

Large Intestine 11 (crease of arm)

Lung 1 (under clavicle)

Stomach 25

Conception Vessel 4 (Tan Den)

Large Intestine 3 (Great Eliminator)

Bladder 40 (backs of knees)

Do not use abdominal, ball of foot, or thumb web positions during pregnancy.

Stomach 36 (below knees) Do Not Use In Pregnancy

Kidney 3 (heels)

Spleen 6 (ankles)

Kidney 3 (heels)

Kidney 1 (balls of feet)

Kidney 1 (balls of feet)

the flow of ki to the legs. This is a good move also for menstrual issues.

Four more pairs of meridian points are located over the bones of the sacrum, the points in the 'holes' of the pelvic spinal bones. These also are for pelvic congestion and good for women with menstrual or reproductive healing issues. The next pair is at the creases where the buttocks meet the legs, and they relax the lower back and hip muscles.

The backs of the knees, small chakra placements, hold a pair of pressure points (and also Reiki positions); the tops of the heels on both sides of the Achilles tendons (hold both sides of each heel at once); and under the center of the foot on the balls of the feet. (Do not use in pregnancy.) Several of these placements are familiar from polarity or from other acupressure sequences. If the woman has varicose veins, make sure not to press on them when working on her legs and feet.

Polarity session neck placements, the Neck Release, or other shiatsu placements may be used for the neck and face. On the front of the body use the PMS emotional sequence point below the clavicle/collarbone to stimulate lung function. Squeeze the points between the thumbs and first fingers of the hands (except in pregnancy). These spots in the webs are a pain release for headaches and toothaches, and they open the sinuses. Squeeze the center of the palm as a calmative for the mind and emotions. Bending her arm, find a tsubo at the outside end of the elbow crease to relieve arm and shoulder pain and to stimulate the large intestine meridian. This is also used in polarity work.

The first abdominal points are on both sides of her navel, about three inches away. Press them toward the navel to stimulate the intestines and relax the abdomen and stomach. The next placement, below the navel, stimulates the whole body and can be done alone. Located on the conception vessel, it corresponds in placement to the belly chakra and is called the hara in Asian healing. Defined as the place where body energy is stored, its cognate is the solar plexus, actually located lower. Press this point with the flat of four fingers deeply, but not causing pain. Avoid the points from abdomen to feet if the woman is pregnant; they stimulate uterine contractions and can cause miscarriage early, but are also helpful later in labor and delivery at term.

The position on the legs is located below the knees, where the two leg bones come together below and outside the knee. The ankle positions are on the inside, four fingers up from the inner ankle bones next to the shins. This pair of pressure points calms and relieves menstrual pain. On the tops of the feet, press one to two inches behind and between the big and second toes on both feet. This point balances the liver meridian. The last points are pairs on the center inside heels, and they stimulate the kidneys. As in other healings, allow the woman to rest at the end of it, keeping her warm and offering her a glass of water when she gets up.

This chapter has been only a beginning of the healing methods of acupressure. For full body sequences and information on specific issues, read the books referenced in this section. Acupressure points are also the needle insertion points for acupuncture, and women interested in one may be drawn to the other. Asian healing is a world of healing in itself.

NOTES

1. Ted Kaptchuk, OMD, *The Web That Has No Weaver: Understanding Chinese Medicine*, (New York, Congdon and Weed, 1983), p. 24.

2. Iona Marsaa Teeguarden, *Acupressure Way of Health: Jin Shin Do*, (New York, Japan Publications, Inc., 1978), p. 8.

3. Merlin Stone, *Ancient Mirrors of Womanhood*, (Boston, Beacon Press, 1984), pp. 24–27.

4. Agency France-Press, "Ancient Feminist Script Found in China," in *The Minneapolis Star Tribune*, Sunday, May 18, 1986.

5. Ted Kaptchuk, *The Web That Has No Weaver*, p. 18.

6. *Ibid.*, p. 35. I will use the Japanese term ki in this chapter, as its connections with Reiki and polarity work are important. Every culture has its own names for this life force energy.

7. *Ibid.*, pp. 38–39.

8. *Ibid.*, p. 20.

9. Iona Marsaa Teeguarden, *Acupressure Way of Health*, pp. 22–26.

10. Ted Kaptchuk, *The Web That Has No Weaver*, p. 53 ff.

11. George W. Meek, Ed., *Healers and The Healing Process*, (Wheaton, Il, Quest/Theosophical Society Books, 1977), pp. 150–155.

12. Ted Kaptchuk, *The Web That Has No Weaver*, p. 77.

13. *Ibid.*, pp. 79–80.

14. Meridians and the elements are from Cathryn Bauer, *Acupressure for Women*, (Freedom, CA, The Crossing Press, 1987), pp. 17–21.

15. *Ibid.*, p. 6.

16. Iona Marsaa Teeguarden, *Acupressure Way of Health*, pp. 88–102, and Lucinda Lidell, *The Book of Massage*, (New York, Simon and Schuster, Inc., 1984), pp. 79–129.

17. Iona Marsaa Teeguarden, *Acupressure Way of Health*, pp. 98–99.

18. Cathryn Bauer, *Acupressure for Women*, pp. 58–60.

19. *Ibid.*, pp. 48–49.

20. *Ibid.*, p. 51.

21. *Ibid.*, p. 118.

22. Mildred Carter, *Body Reflexology*, (West Nyack, NY, Parker Publishing Co., 1983), pp. 47–49.

23. *Ibid.*, pp. 48–49.

24. *Ibid.*, pp. 42–43.

25. *Ibid.*, pp. 182–183.

26. *Ibid.*, pp. 195–197.

27. Lucinda Lidell, *Book of Massage*, (New York, Simon and Schuster, Inc., 1984), p. 129. The shiatsu section is pages 79–129 and is recommended.

Chapter Five

———————◯———————

Foot and Hand Reflexology

Foot and hand reflexology are acupressure based on releasing the seiketsu, the meridian endings, found on the hands and feet. There are 28 seiketsu on the tips of the fingers and toes alone and many more ki channel points on the palms of the hands and soles. The hands and feet are reflecting maps of the body, and by clearing the meridians on them, healing effects are felt in the internal organs. The meridians are the energy channels to the organs, and by releasing blocks (painful areas) in the meridian endings, the healer releases the blocks to ki in the organs themselves.

Reflexology developed from the same Chinese *Nei Jing* roots as acupressure, acupuncture and polarity balancing. It was known in China by about 4000 BCE and in use in Egypt by at least 2330 BCE. A wall painting in the Physician's Tomb in Saqqara, Egypt of that date pictures hand and foot reflexology in practice.[1] The fact that two so geographically separate cultures as China and Egypt share healing knowledge from ancient times, raises again the question of how and when they were in contact. Legends of Atlantis state that Egypt was a colony of that lost continent, and that Atlantean sailors were the ones who did the world travelling. Other sources offer the Phoenicians from later on in time and simultaneous development is also possible. There is no real way to trace the beginnings of the skill, other than to Chinese early writings and the painting in the Egyptian doctor's tomb. Both cultures were healing centers whose teachings spread throughout the world.

An American ear, nose and throat doctor, William H. Fitzgerald, presented his ideas on 'zone therapy' in 1917.[2] He derived his method from extensive study of healing in China and India. His major work divided the body into ten vertical energy zones (used also in polarity balancing), and demonstrated that pressure in one part of a zone could relieve pain or dis-eases located in other parts of it. His zones follow the meridians. A number of medical doctors popularized the idea for awhile, including a Dr. J.S. Riley. In the early 1930s Dr. Riley's assistant, Eunice Ingham learned reflexology from her employer and began to study its effects and to use it. From the early 1930s until her death in 1974, she developed reflexology to what it is today. Ingham emphasized working on the feet, and taught it to enough lay and medical practitioners to establish it. By her many years of study, experiment and teaching, reflexology has been developed into an important healing tool for women. An outgrowth of the complicated theories and methods of Chinese healing, reflexology is a simple and highly effective healing method for the west.

Reflexology is acupressure, and it works in the same ways that acupressure and acupuncture work, following the same principles of Chinese healing. In the theories, energy in the body, the life force ki, travels through twenty channels or meridians (six yin, six yang and eight 'strange flows') that move vertically through the body. The meridians each bring energy to a major organ, are named for their organs, and a clear flow of energy through them is essential for good health. As long as the energy of the meridians is balanced and free flowing, the woman is well. When there is a blockage of ki at any point in a meridian (or zone), however, energy becomes unbalanced with excesses in some points and deficiencies in others, and the block results in dis-ease. Emotional, mental and spiritual dis-ease, as well as physical illness, results from a blockage of ki to any organ or through any meridian. Acupressure, acupuncture, shiatsu, polarity balancing and reflexology all work to release ki blockages in the meridians, thereby opening a free flow of balanced energy and releasing or preventing dis-ease.

A major tool for stress reduction, foot and hand reflexology are also positive techniques for pain relief, muscle relaxation, and an increase in blood circulation and nerve tone. By massaging a tender spot discovered on the foot or hand, pain and dis-ease in internal organs are relieved and healed. Though the practice of reflexology is deceptively simple, its results go deep. A full foot or hand reflexology massage should not be repeated more than once every three or four days, as the release of toxins more quickly can cause disturbing (but not harmful) effects. In self-healing, limit sessions to about ten minutes a day at first. The skill *should not be used in a wanted pregnancy*, as stimulation to some of the meridians can bring on a miscarriage (but can also aid delivery at term). Reflexology should also be avoided for women with varicose veins or phlebitis, and done with care on diabetics, as it can change their insulin balance. For elders, children and pets, the skill is very positive, but use it more gently and less often than with stronger women.

Be aware of the warnings but not put off by them. This is a powerful and positive skill for women's healing, and is especially useful and powerful for self-healing. Reflexology can stop hiccoughs and early migraines, relieve constipation, ease menstrual cramps and pain anywhere in the body, aid childbirth, open stuffed sinuses, help emotional issues, and balance the organs, glands and chakras throughout the body. It can help speed healing and regeneration, speed the release of body toxins, and is positive for virtually every chronic or acute dis-ease or illness. Through the work of Eunice Ingham, reflexology has become widely known in North America and Europe, mainly because it is so simple and effective. It is being taught extensively today by her student Mildred Carter in her several books,[3] and is a system I use personally and recommend.

Reflexology is also a tool for diagnosis. When ki is blocked in an organ, the organ's meridian ending develops a minute granular deposit that the experienced reflexologist feels and works to dissolve. These crystalline deposits are the result of the blockage, and are broken up and dispersed by pressure on the meridian points. Developing the sensitivity to feel these deposits is what makes a woman skilled in reflexology, and takes a lot of practice on a lot of different feet. The woman who knows the map of the organs, allowing for individual differences on each woman she works with, and who can feel these deposits, is able to use reflexology for diagnosis.

A woman who has done reflexology on my feet has done this with me several times, finding dis-eases just beginning or that I had not mentioned. Once it was an early urinary infection, another time a need for new eyeglasses; she has been watching an ovarian cyst that has been there for a couple of years. Pat has saved lives by her ability to diagnose and knows when an illness needs medical care or can be dealt with in self-help. Using massage and finger pressure to break up the granular deposits opens the ki blockage in the meridian, which balances the organ and goes a long way toward dispersing the dis-ease. I have seen this work many times, in this very skilled healer's hands. As in any healing method, if self-help done early and quickly fails, or if the issue is serious, seek medical advice along with alternative methods.

Most healers who use reflexology prefer using the feet to the hands, though the map of the organs is the same for both. The reason for this is in the granular deposits. Women use their hands constantly, and deposits are often dispersed by this. Feet, however, are less flexible and because they are usually protected by shoes, they receive less direct stimulation. Foot reflexes are closer to the surface and the deposits remain for diagnosis. When a woman walks barefoot, especially outdoors, her movements automatically work the reflexes on her soles, probably eliminating dis-ease issues before they manifest. Because most feet are more protected with shoes, they are more likely to keep and show the blockages. Foot reflexology, where the deposits are more readable, is more accurate. When doing an all-over reflexology session more blockages are reached and dispersed in the feet than in the hands. Yet hands are more available at any time for working on and have value in reflexology, too. Both hands and feet are discussed in this chapter, and the woman healer experiments to find the parameters of both.

Pressure used in reflexology is the same as in acupressure but is done differently. The reflex points are under the skin, often against harder bones or muscles, and it takes some probing to find them. When felt, they have the same sharp sensation as when other acupressure points are contacted, a feeling some describe as being like a grain of broken glass. Pressure is applied with thumb or index finger against the point, either in a steady pressure or a massage-type motion. For reflexology covering the whole foot or hand, the basic technique is to work the thumb in a creeping motion up the meridians of the sole and sides of the foot.[4] The movement of the joint makes the forward motion, almost like a caterpillar. The inside edge of the thumb is what makes contact with the skin of the sole or palm—not fingernails or ball of the thumb. The remaining fingers wrap around the woman's foot to steady it. Where a lesser pressure is needed, around the toes for example, use the index finger, moving it in the same creeping motion. This motion differs from other forms of acupressure.

The flesh of the thumb or finger are used, never the nails. I experienced part of a foot reflexology done by a person who insisted on using fingernails. It felt awful, left cuts on my skin, and I refused to allow it to continue. A proper thumb motion, by contrast, feels wonderful and is done without force or pain. The object of reflexology is to release pain areas, not create more of them. Never press so hard that it bruises the skin, either. Correct pressure, thumb and finger movements take practice to develop. Be receptive to the woman's verbal and nonverbal reactions.

Two more specialized movements in reflexology are called hooking and reflex rotation. Hooking is used for tougher places on the feet, as well as for working particularly small or hard to reach pain places. The healer pushes her thumb into the reflex point, then uses a hooking motion to bring it out again, pulling back on the flesh. This takes some practice to learn to do with precision. Reflex rotation is used on highly tender areas to work out painful blockage. It is used only on the lower half of the foot, from heel to the upper abdominal areas (see charts), but not higher on the body map. Holding your thumb on the meridian point, use your other hand to rotate the woman's foot firmly but gently. After a few minutes of rotation, the pain area has usually released. Again, be careful not to use your finger or thumb nails or to work with force.

Reflexology is based on the theories of zone therapy, developed by William Fitzgerald for modern use, but known in ancient Chinese and eastern healing. In this theory, the body is divided into ten vertical zones, energy channels (meridians) through which ki moves through the body in its four directions (ascending, descending, entering and leaving). Horizontally, the energy bands or zones are the ones used in polarity therapy, with the head, torso and legs as the three major divisions. Each organ of the body, following its vertical zone or meridian, is reflected in a place on each of the horizontal divisions, plus on the hands and feet. The ears are another energy map of the body. Therefore, each organ has a reflexing point on head, torso and legs, as well as on hands, feet and ears in its vertical zone.[5]

What this means, is that a sore spot on a woman's left foot, that corresponds on the foot reflexology map to her transverse colon, also gives her sore spots on the same meridians and organ in other portions of her body. Her sore foot point is repeated on both feet, on her left and right hand, on her legs below her knees, on her face, both ears, and on her back.[6] The sore points on her feet are located on the upper parts of neutral charge zones, the almost-center inside edges of her feet. The corresponding sore spots on the other parts of her body are also located on the upper parts of their neutral zone bands, on the inner edges. Though the first sore point is on her left foot, it appears also on her right foot and on both right and left legs and arms.

The ten vertical zones are in five pairs, numbered one to five twice. If there is congestion in one reflex/meridian point on the zone (on the woman's foot, for example), the other sore points are also located on the line of that vertical meridian. The vertical and horizontal sections divide the body into a grid. The zone one pair runs down the center line of the woman's body. One of the pair runs through her left arm, leg and ear, and the other through her right.

Zone Therapy

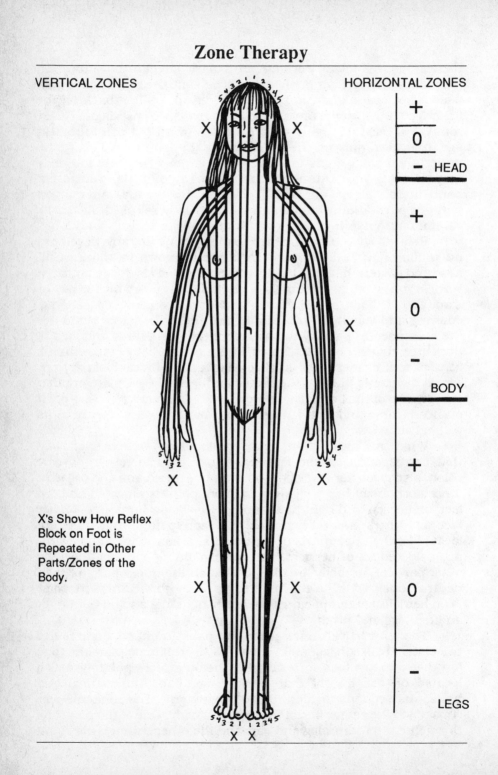

VERTICAL ZONES

HORIZONTAL ZONES

+

0

— HEAD

+

0

—

BODY

+

0

—

LEGS

X's Show How Reflex
Block on Foot is
Repeated in Other
Parts/Zones of the
Body.

Therefore, zone one runs through the woman's thumbs on both sides, her big toes on both sides, and through the inside center line of her body (inside legs, inside arms, inside body and the line on both sides of her spinal column). If there is a blockage on this meridian, blocked meridian points (sore spots) occur all along that zone pair, left and right, one each in every horizontal section of the body. Within the horizontal sections, the points are located on matching energy bands.[7] If her pain area, from the transverse colon and therefore on her torso, is located in a neutral charge zone, other pain spots along the same meridian are also located in neutral charge zones.

With this in mind, the points charted in last chapter's body reflexology illustration are again found on both hands and feet. The scalp also has a body map, as do the ears and tongue, since all of the vertical ki zones run through these organs. The information on energy channels and flows given in the sections on polarity therapy and acupressure all come together in hand and foot reflexology. Yet, when reflexology is taught, the meridians themselves are not emphasized and the meridian points are not identified or numbered. The emphasis is on the body map, that each organ of the body in its relative internal position is mirrored on the soles and toes of the feet, and palms and fingers of the hands. This is a difference in the meridian system that is called reflexology. The other important difference between reflexology and other acupressure or meridian healing skills is in the thumb techniques used to release the points.

The feet and hands themselves are divided into the ten zone therapy vertical zones, five on each foot and hand. The toes and fingers each contain the meridian endings for all five zones, and primarily the thumb and big toe reflex to the head, though all the toes and fingers are used. Horizontally, each foot and hand has the same three energy charge bands that divide other sections of the body, a plus and minus band divided by a neutral zone. In foot reflexology the divisions are named the diaphragm line, waist line and heel line, moving downward from the toes.[8] On the hands, these divisions are also used, though with less emphasis.

The divisions are physical landmarks to look for in doing a reflexology healing. Each woman's feet are slightly different in shape, and the organ map is placed slightly differently on each woman's feet or hands. The energy zones help to find corresponding sore spots on other sections of her body, to be released by finger pressure should she want to do so. Polarity balancing, acupressure and reflexology come together in this process, a mesh of healing methods that are among the oldest healing techniques known. A

Zones on the Feet

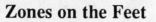

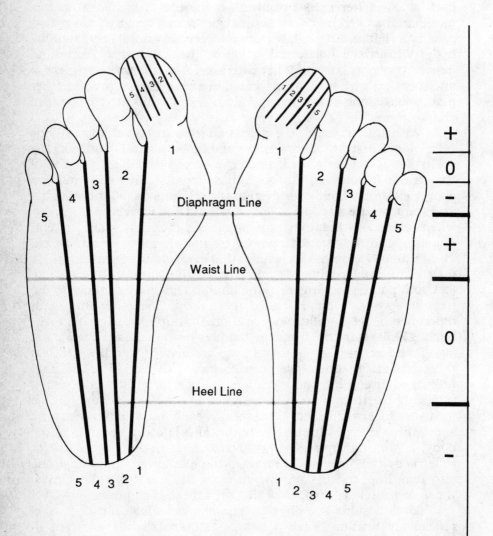

Diaphragm Line

Waist Line

Heel Line

full map of the body is found on the soles of the feet and the palms of the hands, and opening blocks there releases them throughout the woman's body and internal organs.

Hiroshi Motoyama, a healer and physician in Japan who has done electrical work with the chakras and acupressure meridians, has also electrically mapped the meridian endings (seiketsu) in fingers and toes.[9] In his work, he has devised machinery that measures the electrical impulse changes in the endings. With the measurements of his machine, he is able to diagnose dis-ease before it manifests in the physical, much as the reflexologist is able to do by feeling the granular deposits in the meridian endings that are blocked, and that correspond with organs on the organ map of the feet and hands. His work verifies what healers for centuries have known, that when a meridian point is blocked so that its ki flow is decreased or overloaded, pain develops at that spot and later becomes dis-ease in a body organ or part. His electrical measurements also show that

> if we can remove the excessive energy from that point and correct the blockage so that energy can flow smoothly again, then the disease or the subjective symptoms, pain, etc., will disappear.[10]

Many healing skills are based on releasing these blocks to smooth energy flow, in fact every healing skill so far discussed in this book. Perhaps with more research, the medical system will discover what women healers have always known, and begin the alliance between healing and medicine that misogyny has prevented.

The feet and hands are accurate maps of the body's internal organs. By knowing the anatomical location of each major organ, the healer almost knows their locations on the hands and feet. Both feet together (or both hands) are needed to make the full map of woman's body. The spinal column is located on both feet and hands, running along the lines from the edges of the big toes or thumbs down to the heels on the inner sides of the feet or hands. The map for the spine is on both feet or hands placed together, big toe to big toe (or thumb to thumb), with the spine running down the center on both sides, as it runs down the center line of the body. The head is reflexed in the fingers and toes, particularly in the big toes and thumbs, but in all the toes and fingers. The diaphragm line is considered the solar plexus line (on the hands Mildred Carter lists it as the shoulder line), with the lungs above it and the digestive organs below it. The sigmoid colon and sciatic nerve are located below the heel lines.

The reflex to the heart is located in the center of the left sole and palm only (not on both sides), above the diaphragm line, and the liver is located on the right foot or hand only, below the diaphragm line at the little toe or little finger side. If an organ occurs on only one side of the body, that is the one side its reflex is located on. Organs that occur on both sides of the body occur on both sides of the feet and hands. The kidneys, for example, are located one on each side, left side for left kidney, and right side for right kidney. The colon begins on the right sole below the waistline, where it ascends, crosses over to the left sole as it becomes transverse, and descends on the left foot, little toe side from waist to heel. It crosses to the right side of the left sole again for the sigmoid colon and rectum. The pattern is the same on the hands. When locating organs on the map remember that these placements vary slightly from one woman to the next, and also that different reference sources will give slightly different placements for the reflexes on the feet and hands. This is not to say that one source is right and the other is wrong, or that one woman's body map is in the 'wrong places,' only that there are variations. As a woman becomes experienced with reflexology, working on as many feet as she can and doing self-healing, she learns the individual variations. In self-healing she learns what works for her.

Highly important for women, too, are the positions located outside the sole and palm or toes and fingers. These are on the sides of the feet and wrists. The uterus is located below the round protruding bone of the inside ankles, with the ovaries below the outside ankle bones, and the fallopian tubes running across the top of the foot between the ankle bones on the inside and outside. The lymph gland reflex is located at the top of the outer feet, above the round ankle bones. On the inside side of the feet at the archs are the points for the lumbar spine, and behind it on the heels are the placements for the sciatic nerve and to relieve hemorrhoids. The sciatic nerve runs along the Achilles tendon, up the heel.[11] These are mirrored on the wrists, as well. Hand placements for the ovaries are on the little finger sides of the wrists, about two inches down, and the uterus is on the thumb sides of the wrists in the same location. The lower lumbar position is between the ovaries and the hand on the little finger sides, and the one for hemorrhoids is located on the thumb side, between the uterus position and the base of the hand.

Hand and foot positions also correspond with the chakras, based on the reflexology positions for the endocrine system of

Foot Reflexology Body Map

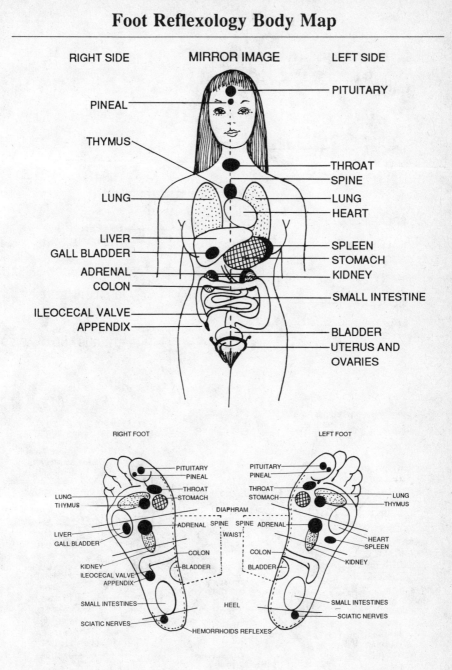

Hand Reflexology Body Map

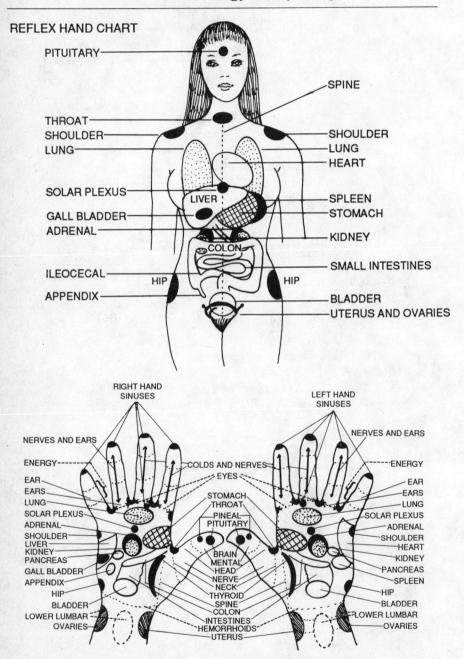

glands.[12] Each ductless or endocrine gland corresponds with a chakra placement and stimulating the glands stimulates and balances each chakra. There are foot and hand placements for each ductless gland, therefore each chakra center. The root center is the uterus (some sources list the adrenals, see below), with foot placements beside the ankle bones on the inside (big toe) side of the feet, or wrists at the thumb sides of the hands. On the wrists, the meridian points are about two inches down. For the belly chakra, the ductless gland is the ovaries, located on the opposite side of the ankle bones (little toe side) and on the little finger sides of the wrists.

The solar plexus is the diaphragm line on the foot, corresponding with the pancreas gland and the adrenals, which are small glands at the top of each kidney. Some designations for the chakras use the adrenals as the root center. The placements for these are between waist and diaphragm lines on the feet, at the centers of the feet, and on the hands also at the centers of the palms. The shiatsu placement with the healer squeezing the centers of the hands was a stimulant for the solar plexus, pancreas and adrenals. The heart chakra is located on the left hand and foot only, and is above the diaphragm, below the second and third toes on the foot, or on the hand running across with the lungs under the second and third fingers. (Some diagrams show the heart as being on the little finger side of the left hand, below the mound of the little finger.) The ductless gland correspondent to the heart chakra is the thymus, which is the body's immune center. Remember the Chinese meridian names for this chakra, the heart and pericardium (heart protector).

At the throat chakra, the ductless gland is the thyroid and parathyroids. The reflexology positions for these glands are above the diaphragm near the insides of the feet, below the big toes. For the hands, the thyroid and parathyroids are on the curve of the thumb creases on the lower palms. The brow chakra or third eye is correspondent to the pituitary gland, the gland that regulates all of the other glands of the body. There is a reflexology spot on the forehead, just at the location of the third eye that reflexes the chakra. On the hands, the reflex meridian point is at the center of the pads of the thumbs and on the feet on the center pads of the big toes. Because these locations are very fleshy, you may have to use deeper pressure to find them.

The crown chakra is associated with the pineal gland, another ductless gland deep in the brain. On the forehead, just above the pressure point for the third eye, there is a reflex point for the crown chakra. On the hands and feet, the reflex meridians are very close

Reflexology for the Chakras

BODY MAP OF THE ENDOCRINE GLANDS

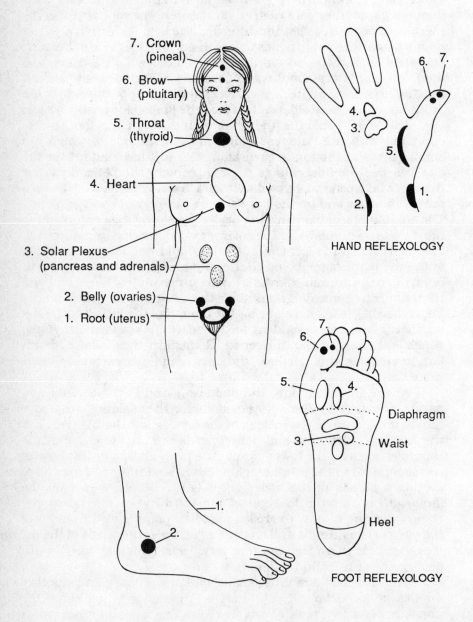

7. Crown
   (pineal)

6. Brow
   (pituitary)

5. Throat
   (thyroid)

4. Heart

3. Solar Plexus
   (pancreas and adrenals)

2. Belly (ovaries)

1. Root (uterus)

HAND REFLEXOLOGY

Diaphragm

Waist

Heel

FOOT REFLEXOLOGY

to the ones for the third eye, on the pads of the thumbs and big toes. Press deeply for them.

Stimulating the meridians that access the chakras is a way of chakra balancing and of stimulating a woman's entire Natural Ki. The thymus, heart center, is particularly important to work with in case of any illness or infection, as its output balances the body's full immune system. For persons with AIDS, arthritis, multiple sclerosis, asthma, allergies or cancer—dis-eases resulting from immune system failure or overreaction (deficiency or excess of ki), pay particular attention to the thymus. The pituitary and pineal glands activate and regulate all of the other hormone-producing ductless glands, and are important to keep free flow of ki. In women's menstrual cycle or hormonal imbalances, be sure to stimulate them, and in any dis-ease of any endocrine gland. The thyroid, throat chakra, regulates the body's metabolism, and the tiny parathyroids that are stimulated with them affect mental and physical stability. The solar plexus/pancreas is vital for digestion and the distribution of ki and nutrition through the body. The uterus and ovaries are women's reproductive system and their hormones function in women's menstrual cycles and hormonal balance. When stimulating these centers for specific dis-eases also stimulate the pituitary and pineal glands (brow and crown chakras). The adrenals, above the kidneys, are survival drive and energy. A reflexology session that works to open blocks to these ductless glands balances the chakras and aids women's well-being.

Now begin a full foot reflexology session, stimulating all the foot meridians and using pressure/massage on every part of the body map.[13] The description is for working with another woman, but is variable for self-use. Refer to the material given earlier on the creeping thumb technique. Do one foot completely before moving to the other one, either foot first, and begin at the top of the foot, with the toes. The toes on the body map reflex the head, with the big toes as head, brain and neck, and the smaller toes as the sinuses at the tips and the senses at the bases (eyes and ears below the lowest toe joints). If you are using the left foot, support the toes with the right hand, using your left thumb to apply pressure to the reflexes, and bracing the foot with the other fingers of the left hand. On the right foot, work in the opposite manner. Walk your thumb along each toe to the base, beginning with the big toe, and returning at the end from the other side. The toes are small, and it takes some practice to get the feel of the thumb motion. If by your touch or the woman's response you find a tender spot, apply pressure to release it.

Then use the same creeping thumb motion horizontally across

the fleshy pad at the base of the toes, changing thumbs at the end and repeating in both directions. Remember to use the sides, rather than the balls of the thumbs to do this, and avoid using fingernails. Work the neck and throat reflex next, at the base of the big toe. This is also for the tonsils, top of spine, and the thyroid and parathyroid glands. Work around the base of the big toe from the side, changing hands to do the other side, and supporting the foot with the hand not being used.

Next, beginning at the bottom of the ball of the foot, work the thumb in a creeping motion between the metatarsal joints, from the bottom of the ball to the toe bases and back down again. Do this all the way across the foot, changing hands at the top and bottom of each row. The movement is a pinching one using the thumb on the sole of the foot, the index finger held behind it on the top of the foot. Hold the toes in the other hand, and cover the area thoroughly. Then use your index finger to work the same reflexes, this time on the top, rather than on the sole. Reflexes on this upper part of the foot, above the diaphragm line, are for the lungs, shoulders, heart and respiratory system.

Returning to the sole of the foot, the next reflexes are for the upper and lower abdominal areas. The upper abdominal area concentrates on the liver, and is located running between the ball of the foot (metatarsal line, diaphragm line) and the waist line. Use the thumbs to work up and down the entire area in vertical lines, changing hands at the top and bottom, and using the opposite hand to support the foot at the toes. For the right foot, use hooking to reach the reflex for the ileocecal valve and appendix, in the lower abdominal area on the little toe side. Walk your thumb from this point to the waist line. For the ascending colon (right foot), walk up the foot, and for the descending colon (left foot, outer side), walk down it. The ascending colon releases issues of some digestive disorders, bronchitis, asthma and allergies. The descending colon reflexes such disorders as constipation and gas, migraines, and other stress reaction issues. The sigmoid colon is below the heel line, on the tough-skinned heel of the lower foot, and requires heavier pressure to contact.

The spine is next, worked in a continuous thumb movement from heel to toes, on the big toe sides of both feet. Each curve in the foot matches a curve in the spine, and working the spinal foot reflexes aids relaxation and release of muscle tension throughout the body. You will need to move your hand at least once to do this, moving the supporting fingers from around the foot. Support the foot at the toes with your other hand, and with the fingers of the hand you are using as you apply pressure. The skin at the heel is tougher and requires more pressure, but it thins as you move up. If you contact any tender spots, apply massaging pressure, but if the woman has a chronically bad back, don't try to 'cure' it in one session. The rule here is to apply pressure three times with released pressure in between, then go on.

For hips, knees and legs (again on both feet, but do one foot at a time), the reflex runs along the side of the foot, just above the spinal line on the little toe side. The hip reflex moves to the back of the ankle joint and is also the sciatic nerve point. Hold the foot upright with your supporting hand, and with your working hand use thumb or index finger to walk across all parts of the area, covering it thoroughly in all directions. Again, if there are sore spots, try to work them out with pressure or massage. Work along the heel up to the ankle, across the top of the ankle, and above and below the round ankle bones. These movements reflex the lower back, hips, knees, sciatic nerves, uterus and ovaries. Working along the top of the foot, between the round protruding bones on the sides, also massages the fallopian tubes. Change to the other foot and repeat.

The preceding process covers every area of the body map, and therefore every organ. If you hit a tender spot, check the charts to see what organ the spot reflexes. For self-healing, Mildred Carter suggests using the knuckle of the index finger to apply pressure on the centers of the feet, the abdominal areas, and suggests particular attention to the stomach areas to heal ulcers. She offers a warning to diabetics, that reflex massage to the pancreas/solar plexus can increase the body's natural insulin production, upsetting the balance of insulin medication. Be aware of this and take measures in case of possible shock.[14] In heart conditions, the woman receiving the healing can feel very well after it. The warning here is not to over-exert because she feels better, but to continue taking it easy until complete healing has taken place.[15] In any reflexology treatment, make sure to do both feet. The positions are given from the viewpoint of one woman working on another, the soles of the woman's feet facing the healer. Self-healing is also encouraged with foot reflexology, bend your knee to rest your foot on your lap or beside your hip to reach all of the positions and massage the whole foot. Don't forget to do the sides of the feet, backs of the heels, and around the ankle bones.

Mildred Carter describes a quicker way of doing reflexology as self-healing, using a variety of special tools. Her primary one for the feet looks like a rubber dumbbell with short spokes in the center, and for the hands a ball with rubber spokes or nubs protruding from it. Another foot tool looks somewhat like a bent pizza cutter, to apply pressure in hard to reach places. For the hands she also uses a metal or wooden shatterproof wide-toothed comb to apply pressure by holding down on it, and wooden clamps like clothespins for the finger tips. These tools are available from some health centers and healthfood stores. The warning is not to leave the clamps on so long as to harm circulation and not to overdo it. The tools release a lot of meridian points just by squeezing and playing with them, or by rotating them underfoot. Work with them for about ten minutes at a time only every other day at first.[16] This is important since overdoing releases more toxins into the system than the body can handle easily at one time. No harm will come of it, but why feel the effects? This is an especial caution for elders and women who are debilitated or weakened by their healing issues. Again, never use pressure on injuries or broken bones, and avoid reflexology of hands or feet in pregnancy to prevent early contractions and miscarriage.

Hand reflexology is basically the same as working on the feet, with the body map in the same places, and the hand motions similar.[17] The hands are shorter and wider than the feet, so the body map is slightly different. The hands get a lot more use and exercise than the feet, and are bonier surfaces with the reflexes deeper, so that feeling the granular deposits and sore spots is harder to do. Reflexologists in general find better results working with the feet, but the hands contain the same reflexes and body map and are available to work on at any moment. If a woman has varicose veins and is unable to use foot reflexology, her hands are another working source. In self-healing, if a woman is unable to bend her legs to positions she can reach with her hands, or is unable to move her legs to use the massage tools, hand reflexology is still open to her. In another note for disabled women, if a limb, finger or toe has been amputated, the reflex spots in it are still accessible at the end of the stump.[18] In hand reflexology, use your thumbs to work the palms of the hands, and your index fingers between the fingers and on the hand backs. As with the feet, avoid using pressure on a broken limb or over broken skin or a bruise.

In hand reflexology, again use the thumb in a creeping motion to massage all the surface of the palms. The process is the same, transferred from the foot sequence to the map of the hands. Massage each finger thoroughly, with thumb and first finger in a pinching motion, looking for sore spots along the sides and backs of the joints and around the fingernails. In the lung reflexes, as with the feet, work your thumb up and down the inside of the hand, then go to the back of the hand, working in a line from between the fingers down to the ends of the hollows between the bones. The spinal reflexes are more accessible than most of the hand reflexes, so massage them thoroughly from the tip of the thumb to below the wrist. Don't forget to use pressure on the uterus, ovaries, lymph and lower spinal points on the wrists below the hands, and remember to do both hands.

The web between the thumbs and first fingers is an area not easily correspondent in foot reflexology. Shiatsu calls this meridian point 'the great eliminator' for its versatile ability to relieve many kinds of pain and congestion. Use a pinch and roll technique to massage the entire area of the webs on both hands. It relieves stuffed sinuses, hiccoughs, headache and migraine pain, toothaches, and any other sort of pain. The web includes reflexes to the throat, neck, spine, stomach, thyroid, liver (right hand) and heart (left hand). Apply pressure to the tips of all the fingers for pain in general, and work the webs between the other fingers (and on the toes).[19]

Other hand and foot reflexes to use for **pain** are the pineal and pituitary points on the pads of the thumbs and big toes, a horizontal line running across the heel lines of both soles, and the centers of the feet just below the diaphragm lines. There is a spot on thumbs and big toes at the lower edges of the nails that is a pain relief spot, plus a row of spots below the joints of the second and third fingers and toes on the backs of the hands and tops of the feet. Look for one more below the bones of the ankles, the little round protruding bone on the big toe side. All of these points cause the release of endorphins from the brain, natural pain-inhibiting chemicals. Also try the lower legs along the shin bones, at the bottoms of the calf muscles; there are several pain points there, on the big toe sides of the legs.[20] Some of these were used in acupressure sequences. If any of these points feels tender, massage the pain.

An interesting use of wooden or metal combs (I prefer wooden ones) in hand reflexology is in **childbirth** labor and delivery. The technique can bring the baby on quickly and should not be started before labor begins, and only in a safe place to deliver. The directions are to use a comb for each hand, not plastic ones that could shatter, holding the comb teeth down against the palms, pressing steadily and continuously with the fingers on them during contractions. Hold until the hands get tired, then relax and hold again. This relieves the pain of contractions, speeding the dilation process in the first stage and speeds delivery in the second stage. The urge to grasp something is an instinct in laboring women, and by pressing the reflexes, pain is lessened and the labor is speeded up measurably. Don't experiment with this during pregnancy, as it can bring on labor (or a miscarriage if too early). Wait for labor to start and try it only in a safe place to deliver.[21] Commercial reflexology combs have thick teeth with rounded ends to prevent damage to the hands.

To bring on **menstruation**, use the reflexes of the tongue. The tongue, like the ears, is another organ that contains all of the ten vertical zones. Using a tongue depressor or the handle of a tablespoon, press the tongue as far back as you can without gagging in a firm steady pressure. Hold for two to three minutes, then relax, and move the pressure from the center to one side, then to the other side of the back of the tongue position. This will bring on menstruation quickly, sometimes immediately. Relieve menstrual pain by the same method, holding the spoon or tongue depressor about two-thirds of the way back. Meridian zones one, two and three are pressed. The technique is safe to do every month. Use hand pressure on the thumbs and first two fingers, as well.[22]

For **hot flashes**, work on all of the positions of the endocrine glands, on hands, feet or body, as well as the positions for the ovaries and uterus. Pay particular attention to reflexes of the ovaries and pituitary glands. In epilepsy, also, work with the endocrine gland reflexes.[23] For constipation work the reflexes of the ascending, transverse and descending colon, plus the sigmoid colon, the organs of the lower abdomen.

Reflexology has a variety of treatment techniques for **headaches**, since headaches and migraines are caused by a variety of causes. First, work with the reflexes on and between all of the fingers or toes, particularly the thumb or big toe and particularly the web between the thumb and first finger (or big toe and first toe). Massage all the joints thoroughly on the fingers and toes, sides, fronts and backs of the fingers from tips to base. When you find tender spots you are on the right track; massage them out. Also work on the pads of the palms and feet below the toe joints, since the dis-ease could be coming from neck tension. Try the reflexes for the stomach, as many headaches come from digestive disturbances, and for the colon. Work on the thumb and big toe, the upper spinal/neck reflexes and along the spine points of hands or feet. In relieving headaches with reflexology, start with the thumbs or big toes, then move to the next fingers or toes, until you find the sore spots to concentrate on.[24]

In working with **hypoglycemia**, low blood sugar, reflex the meridians to all of the endocrine glands/chakras, and pay particular attention to the pancreas, thymus and adrenals. Work the reflexes to the liver, as well.[25] Use hands or feet for this (feet are considered more successful), and do it frequently (a couple of times a week). Work out any sore spots as you find them. Hypoglycemia is a problem for a large number of women, and is considered by some practitioners to be a pre-diabetic state. High protein, low sugar diets are recommended, and frequent small meals.

If you are working with a woman (or yourself) who has a **bad back**, reflexing the spinal column meridians can be a great help in relieving pain and easing movement. Use either hand or foot reflexology, the spinal reflexes on the hands are more accessible than some of the other hand reflexes, and work out sore spots thoroughly. If a spot is too tender, go to the other foot or hand as it may be less tender, then go back to the original pain point. If the woman is in a great deal of back pain, it may be best to do the rest of the reflex massage first, and go to the spinal meridians after she is fully relaxed by the rest of the massage. Do not try to relieve years of pain or structural problems in one sitting. Work a sore spot for a time, then go on to another spot, and do another reflexology treatment in a few days. Reflexology on the pain areas and spinal meridians will not correct structural defects, but reflexology relieves pain and muscle tension.[26] Suggest that the woman also see a chiropractor, and do reflexology along with it. With spinal issues, do whole body reflexology often, rather than working only on the spine.

With **arthritis, AIDS, multiple sclerosis, cancer** or any debilitating dis-ease, work in reflexology beginning with the endocrine glands, the chakra system. Pay special attention here to the pituitary gland and thymus (in arthritis to the adrenals), but massage thoroughly to stimulate all of the chakra reflexes and all of the endocrine system glands. When this is done, go over the hands or feet thoroughly, massaging all of the reflexes and looking for pain spots. Work on any pain spots you find, massaging them out if possible. If a spot is too tender, try working it on the other foot or hand, or doing what you can with it, then going on to other areas for a few minutes. Come back to the pain spot and try again. Plan to do a full foot massage about every other day, but make the first ones very gentle, particularly if there is a great deal of pain or the woman is very debilitated. The endocrine sequence is a great help in rejuvenation and healing, and releasing pain spots can go a long way toward relieving internal/body pain.[27] Even if the dis-ease is terminal, reflexology can give a great deal of relief. For many dis-eases that seem terminal but are not, reflexology can turn the course around by returning a free flow of ki through the meridians and organs.

Multiple sclerosis is an increasing issue among women with much more healing research needed. Like AIDS or arthritis, it is a dis-ease of the immune system, and increasing thymus/heart chakra action, plus pituitary/third eye function with reflexology is helpful. Try Reiki or polarity balancing along with reflexology massage.

Use the reflexes in the web between the thumbs and first fingers (or big and first toes) to open the sinuses in **colds**. Since colds are an elimination process of the immune system, it is not positive to use reflexology (or medicine's over-the-counter drugs) to try to stop them. Reflexology releases more toxins into the system for the body to eliminate. Work briefly on the lung and kidney meridian points to speed the elimination process. For sore throats and tonsilitis, massage under the big toes or around the thumbs. Use massage on the thumbs and first and second fingers (or big toe and first and second smaller ones) for coughs. Use the tongue reflexes, pressed with a spoon handle or tongue depressor in the center of the tongue for five to ten minutes. Also try pressing the thumb against the lower joint of the first finger to stop a cough. In cases of fevers, again a way of combating dis-ease by the immune system, do reflexology only when the fever has gone on too long or goes too high. Press the reflexes of the pituitary and pineal glands (brow and crown chakras) in the pads of the thumbs or big toes.[28]

Holding the fingers tip to tip and pressing on them is a reflexology way of relieving **nervous tension and insomnia**. The tips of the toes work, too, but it is harder to do this. The trick is to place pressure on all of the finger or toe tips at once. Pressing hands together is one way of doing it, or using reflexology clamps that look like clothespins (or clothespins themselves) to press on the fingers. If using clamps or other artificial means of placing pressure, make sure to take them off after a few minutes, before the fingers turn blue.[29] Be very careful not to cut off circulation. In cases of tension and exhaustion, a full reflexology session, massaging the surfaces of both hands or feet, does wonders—far more than reflexing one point only. For another single point, try working with the crown chakra points of the pineal gland, on the pads of the thumbs and big toes.

In one more healing sequence from Mildred Carter, there are reflexology moves to use for **heart dis-ease**, and can be used in an attack while waiting for professional help. The reflex point here is to massage the pad under the little finger of the left hand with the thumb of the right. This can also be done by massaging under the little toe of the left foot. Massage all of the area of the left hand or foot in the placement of the heart and lungs, the whole little finger or little toe side of the upper hand or foot. Work on any reflex that is tender and continue across the hand or foot to the thumb or big toe. Do this regularly, not only in pain or emergencies. For high blood pressure, work the liver reflexes and the pituitary gland meridians, and do a full hand or foot reflexology session about twice a week. Carter reports that using reflexology on stroke patients may help them to regain full or fuller movement and recovery.[30]

With careful use, reflexology is a very important women's healing method. Like several more complicated healing systems, it opens the blocks that prevent free flow of life force energy and stimulates the healing of dis-ease. It increases circulation, nerve tone, reduction of stress, and stimulates regeneration and the effects of the immune, lymphatic and endocrine systems. The skill has been known since very ancient times worldwide and has proved then and now to be effective and positive. Most women learn to do it for themselves or others readily. For women unable to apply the pressure required manually, there are massaging tools on the market or that can be devised at home to help. While reflexology is not to be used by women in pregnancy or on the feet with varicose veins, and in diabetes only carefully, many, many women can benefit from it. Reflexology is useful on even the youngest children, on elders and on pets. No tools or few tools are required. The thumb and finger pressure movements take a bit of practice but are fairly simple to learn, and the map of the body is far less involved than the meridian points of other meridian systems.

NOTES

1. Lucinda Lidell, *The Book of Massage*, (New York, Simon and Schuster, Inc., 1984), pp. 13 and 130.

2. *Ibid.* Mildred Carter, in her book, *Helping Yourself with Foot Reflexology*, (W. Nyack, NY, Parker Publishing Co., 1969), p. 1 gives the date as 1913.

3. Mildred Carter, *Body Reflexology, Helping Yourself With Foot Reflexology*, and *Hand Reflexology: Key to Perfect Health*, (W. Nyack, NY, Parker Publishing Co., 1983, 1969 and 1975 respectively). Much of this chapter follows her work.

4. Lucinda Lidell, *The Book of Massage*, pp. 138–139.

5. Richard Gordon, *Your Healing Hands*, (Santa Cruz, CA, Unity Press, 1978), pp. 19 and 96 ff.

6. *Ibid.*, p. 96.

7. Lucinda Lidell, *The Book of Massage*, p. 132.

8. *Ibid.*, p. 133.

9. George W. Meek, Ed., *Healers and the Healing Process*, (Wheaton, IL, Quest/Theosophical Book Society, 1977), pp. 153–155.

10. *Ibid.*, p. 155.

11. Mildred Carter, *Body Reflexology*, (W. Nyack, NY, Parker Publishing Co., 1983), p. 32.

12. *Ibid.*, pp. 30 and 116–125.

13. Lucinda Lidell, *Book of Massage*, pp. 140–145. The same material is found in Mildred Carter, *Helping Yourself With Foot Reflexology*, p. 21 ff.

14. Mildred Carter, *Helping Yourself With Foot Reflexology*, p. 68.

15. *Ibid.*, pp. 80–81.

16. *Ibid.*, p. 24, and *Hand Reflexology: Key to Perfect Health*, (W. Nyack, NY, Parker Publishing Co. 1975), pp.68–86. Reflexology tools are available from Stirling Enterprises, Inc., Box 216, Cottage Grove, OR, 97424, write for catalog.

17. Hand sequence is based on Lucinda Lidell, *Book of Massage*, pp. 146–148, with additional material from Mildred Carter, *Hand Reflexology: Key to Perfect Health*, p. 51 ff.

18. Mildred Carter, *Hand Reflexology: Key to Perfect Health*, p. 218.

19. *Ibid.*, p. 62.

20. Mildred Carter, *Body Reflexology*, p. 34.

21. Mildred Carter, *Hand Reflexology: Key to Perfect Health*, pp. 210–215.

22. *Ibid.*, pp. 206–207.

23. Mildred Carter, *Helping Yourself With Foot Reflexology*, pp. 135–136, and p. 16.

24. Mildred Carter, *Hand Reflexology: Key to Perfect Health*, pp. 97–100.

25. *Ibid.*, pp. 138–140.

26. Mildred Carter, *Helping Yourself With Foot Reflexology*, pp. 41–47.

27. *Ibid.*, pp. 148–151.

28. Mildred Carter, *Hand Reflexology: Key to Perfect Health*, pp. 166–170.

29. *Ibid.*, pp. 232–233.

30. *Ibid.*, pp. 115–121.

Chapter Six

—————————○—————————

Pendulums, Muscle Testing and Applied Kinesiology

Using a pendulum is very different from doing reflexology, acupressure, polarity balancing, Reiki or laying on of stones, but it still uses ki energy. The seemingly simple skill of the pendulum becomes the slightly more advanced one of muscle testing, and the very advanced one of applied kinesiology. All are forms of using ki/ Goddess-within life force energy for women's healing. The pendulum is a simple tool for making choices, which works by reflection of the ki flowing from within. Muscle testing uses the body itself as the tool for the same purpose. Applied kinesiology is a very complicated form of muscle testing and release used primarily by chiropractors, reflecting the meridian information used by acupressure and acupuncture. All three methods use ki to help women make clear choices about their health, what will benefit them and what will not. This chapter introduces these three skills, from simple pendulums to the most difficult, applied kinesiology.

The material in this section is a bridge between the bodywork skills of the first half of this book, and the ki-from-within essences of the rest of it. Where the skills of the first five chapters worked with energy by influencing the aura from the outside, the next four work by influencing women's ki from within, using vitamins, and minerals, herbs, homeopathy, flower essences and gemstone elixirs for women's health and well-being. There are a multitude of possible choices in these chapters, and a woman decides which (or which combination) of the many possibilities is right for her. More specifically, she decides which of many good choices is the best for her own needs at a particular place and time. Pendulums or muscle testing are helpful tools. They combine psychic and medical skill, and can be surprisingly accurate when used correctly and with common sense. Muscle testing is probably more accurate than the pendulum, while applied kinesiology in skilled hands is highly so. These are important women's tools for diagnosis and healing.

Modern medicine makes the patients fit their treatments, rather than fitting the treatment to the woman. Medicine gives women its high rate of iatrogenic dis-eases and unnecessary surgeries. Women's healing, by contrast, raises women's quality of life and well-being by its focus on the woman herself. Medicine is misogynist and women's healing is gynist. An increasing number of women MD's are trying to change this stance, but their percentage is small and change is slow. Any system or treatment that does not honor women's bodies and Being is misogynist (including some that call themselves New Age), but medicine is built on misogyny.

When a woman goes to a doctor and tells him her problem, he ignores her and takes $1000 worth of tests, then tells her what she already told him was wrong. When a woman works with a woman healer in mutual cooperation, the two women learn together what is wrong, going primarily by the woman's own body knowledge, and they choose together how to help her. Women in self-healing work to get well, mainly by taking power and going within for knowledge.

The major differences between medicine and healing are in the choices and who makes and implements them. When a woman goes to any but the most exceptional doctor, it's the doctor who does all the choosing and deciding. He may choose for her a drug that makes her sicker than she was before, not weighing its side effects (or not asking her to weigh them) against her quality of life. When she reacts with discomfort, there is nothing the doctor can do for her (unless he gives her more drugs to counteract the first one), and he often doesn't care. Herbalists, Chinese traditional medicine and homeopathy all recognize that a drug's side effects are part of its effects. There is no separating a drug's positive and negative actions. The doctor may tell the woman she needs surgery, not because she truly needs it, but because it costs more, or because it's the easiest way for him to 'cure' her, or because it's the popular method for her dis-ease this year. The woman has no choices in the medical system; the doctor decides for her on the basis of what he wants to do, not on the basis of her real needs.

> When the public spends $5,200,000,000 for prescription drugs and another $2,200,000,000 for non-prescription drugs a year and they don't need two-thirds of them, it is time we take stock of what is going on in the health field.[1]

It's the doctor, not the woman, who implements the choices for these drugs and surgeries, and the woman who takes the consequences.

In women's healing, the woman decides herself what treatment or healing method, or no method, she accepts. She is informed of all the possibilities, with no information withheld, and picks one or more methods that she feels best fit her needs. She works with the healer to understand the parameters and possibilities of each healing system. There are no drugs with side effects, no surgeries except as a very last resort, usually only when her issue is too advanced. The women discuss the positive and negative aspects of each method, its cost (which in women's healing should be negligible), the time it takes, what it involves, and how it fits the woman's needs and lifestyle. There may be a combination of methods or ideas for the woman to choose from—diet, herbs, reflexology, Reiki, polarity, vitamins, etc. Within each method there is a series of choices—exactly how to use it, how much and how often, which and in what combinations.

The woman fits the methods to her own healing needs, and, as her healing progresses, her body changes and her requirements may change. The herb that worked well for her last month has completed its use and now she needs something different. The homeopathic remedy that helped at the beginning has stopped helping her or her symptoms may have changed. The diet[2] that was satisfying and healthy, that gave her additional well-being three months ago, leaves her less satisfied now. The vitamins that made a difference have changed her needs. The woman and the healer or the woman alone make many choices at each step, fitting the treatment to the woman's healing. This is the major difference between medicine and women's healing—that the woman has the choices, control and implementation of her healing in her own hands, and that the treatment fits her individually.

To make her various choices, the woman starts with information. She reads, talks with other women about the methods, compares their healing issues with her own, and meditates or looks within to her guides or Goddess-within for help. She talks to a healer, someone outside herself, who may have different information or more experience to offer her, or more objectivity or skill, but the decisions are still her own. She works with a lot of conscious information and learns methods to tap her subconscious, to ask her Goddess-within, her aura self, what her body needs. A pendulum, muscle testing, or applied kinesiology help her to access that inner woman for nonconscious information about her health. The answers are all inside her.

When I do individual healing work, some time in the course of the trancework, Reiki or laying on of stones, I ask her, "Where did this come from?" At least ninety percent of women know and tell me. If I ask her the same question in a conscious, daily life state, I get few answers. In the highly relaxed, meditative state of deep healing, the woman knows. Then I ask her, "What do you need for healing to happen?" And again she almost always knows, and I help her in any way I can to have what she needs for her healing. If she doesn't know, I tell her to go to a place inside her and ask her Goddess-within. The answer comes. It sounds simple, and it usually is.

A pendulum or muscle testing is a method and tool by which women reach the information that is there within them without my questioning them. Pendulums are divination tools, and divination means to bring information from the subconscious to the conscious surface. This is what happens in a tarot reading, when all the appropriate, meaningful cards come up in the layout, or in an I Ching reading, when the randomly thrown coins draw a written hexagram that gives a woman the advice she needs. A pendulum can be used to ask specific questions and gain specific advice, but it is not an oracle. It is particularly valuable in healing issues, healing questions and choices, because the subconscious that it taps into is intimately aware of what it needs. If the subconscious can send bad metaphors of healing issues (as when 'give me a break' manifests into a broken leg), it can also send more positive ones of how to heal what may be out of balance in a woman's life. The subconscious is the emotional body aura level, and the pendulum as a tool is a means of divining information from the woman's emotional body within.

Physically, a pendulum is a very simple thing. It's an object of slight weight (in a variety of types and shapes) swinging on the end of a string or chain. My pendulum is an eleven-inch length of silver necklace chain, longer than those most women use, with a crystal at one end and a tumbled peridot gemstone at the other. I have used any necklace I wear as a pendulum at one time or another and have been pleased with the results, but a ring or button on a string also works. Some women are very fussy about the type of pendulum they use, while others use anything. Some women spend a lot of money for carved silver weights, and others swear that only a lucite pointed cylinder is accurate. Yet all get what they need from the pendulums they choose. Lengths of chain (or cord or string) vary from a few inches to over a foot, and the type of pendants vary just as much. Obviously it isn't the physical property of the pendulum itself that is important.

Egyptian cave paintings, discovered in 1949 in the Atlas Mountains, depict a dowser searching for water. The paintings of the Caves of Tassili have been Carbon 14 tested and found to be 8000 years old. Finding water was a survival skill to a desert people. The dowsing rod is the foremother of the pendulum. Dowsing with a divining rod and dowsing with a pendulum are the same skill, known everywhere in ancient times, in the same diversity of cultures and geographies familiar to other healing skills. Dowsing and pendulums were known to the Egyptians, Hebrews, Scythians, Persians, Medes, Etruscans, Druids, Greeks, Romans, Hindus, Chinese, Polynesians, Peruvians and Native Americans.[3] Artifacts from 1300 BCE in Mesopotamia, and 2200 BCE in China show dowsing and dowsing tools, as well as in ancient Africa, and in India throughout its history. Wherever there was mining, dowsing and pendulums were standard equipment throughout the world from very ancient to modern times. The pendulum or dowsing rod was used to locate metals as well as water. By the middle ages in Europe, the rod had become the swinging pendulum, and the skill became known as radiesthesia. By its antiquity, it was surely known to the matriarchies, and its knowledge was carried among the same cultures in the ways other forms of healing were communicated. Women everywhere today have reclaimed this simple tool, probably reintroduced by crystal workers.

To begin using a pendulum, first make or obtain one. The materials for it can be simple household things. I prefer a crystal on the end of mine and recommend it, but when using gemstones as pendulums, it becomes important to keep the stones cleared. I place mine in dry sea salt or under a pyramid every few days to clear it; if the stones become too overloaded with energies, they stop registering or throw some very wild responses. Try different lengths for the chain or cord between the pendulum and holding knob. Some women feel that metal for this deflects the energies, but I feel it enhances them; try and see what works for you. The knob at the end is usually smaller than the pendulum itself and comfortable to hold.

Once you have made the pendulum and cleared the stones (if they are gemstones), begin working with it. Hold it by the knob and let it swing for a moment. Hold it with thumb and first two fingers on the knob, so that a neutral (thumb), minus (index finger) and plus (middle finger) energy charge all contact the tool at once. Most women receive energy from their left hand and send it from their right, but a few are the opposite. If you send energy from your right hand, that is the hand to hold the pendulum in. By holding it in the receiving hand, it only swings randomly. If you hold the pendulum in your right hand and pass the palm of your left underneath it, the pendulum reacts, mine with a No, to the electrical energy of your palm. I get the same No holding it in my receiving hand. Other women may react differently.

Once you get the feel of the pendulum and have determined which is your sending hand, establish its code, the means by which it connects you to your inner Being. A pendulum has six possible ways of moving, up and down, side to side, circularly clockwise or counter-clockwise. It can also swing randomly or just hover in place. With a shorter cord or chain, the pendulum is more likely to give a circular response pattern; with a longer one it moves up and down. As you hold your pendulum in your sending hand, your other hand away from it, clear your mind and concentrate on thinking, "Give me a Yes" and watch what the pendulum does. Continue thinking Yes, and become familiar with what the pendulum's Yes looks like. For most women it's a circular, clockwise pattern or an up and down one.

Then, in the same way concentrate on thinking, "Give me a No" and watch the change in movement. If the pattern was circular, it may go up and down, or become circular in the opposite direction. If it was an up and down pattern, the swing might change to right and left. When you are clear on what the No looks like, alternate on thinking Yes and No at it and watching the patterns shift. Another way is to hold the pendulum over a minus finger (index) and ask for a No, over a plus finger (middle) and ask for a Yes, and over the neutral thumb and ask for a Maybe. In a few minutes of this, you will know what means Yes and No on your pendulum.

For many years I was unable to use a pendulum to give me meaningful answers, though I tried several different ones at intervals. Being dyslexic, the circular patterns I got with them were clear to everyone but me. If it circled from left to right as a Yes and right to left as a No, (which is what it did), both directions looked the same and I couldn't identify the answers. I depended a lot on a friend who had better success but who got tired of being called on the phone all the time to help. Finally, I decided to make my own pendulum, something I hadn't tried before, and to ask it to give me a Yes and No I could easily read. I made my present long-chained model and in establishing the codes requested patterns clear to me. For a Yes I got a long up and down swing, and for a No a circular one. I keep it with me at all times and use it extensively now.

Once you have determined Yes and No on your pendulum, it

takes a bit of time to connect your conscious and subconscious mind. A pendulum can only answer Yes and No questions, and possibly by its non-answer give a Maybe. Take something familiar in your hand, your daily vitamin perhaps, and ask it, "Is this my vitamin?" Ask it a number of very obvious yes and no questions over a period of a few days. Using the energy charges you know from polarity work, touch or hold the object you are asking about with your left (receiving) hand, while holding the pendulum in your right (sending) hand. Make sure you are holding the knob with all three fingers, so there is a plus, minus and neutral charge going through the pendulum. The answers are steadier and clearer for doing this.

Your aura is the electrical energy directing the Yes and No of the pendulum, so when your energy is off, your pendulum is off too. If you are very tired, the pendulum becomes inaccurate. If you don't feel well, it may be erratic, more so if you are angry or upset. If you want something a lot, don't ask the pendulum if you should have it—you'll always get a Yes. If you don't want something but think you should do it, the pendulum follows your emotions and gives you a No. If your body's energy lines are crossed, by sitting with your legs crossed for example, the pendulum gets confused. Some women feel that a pendulum is inaccurate in electrical storms.[4] You receive the clearest pendulum answers when your mind is clear and in an alpha state, and when your emotions are neutral, since your own aura energy, your subconscious/emotional body, directs the information that it gives you.

The subconscious/emotional body also can answer only when it has the necessary information. If you ask it about a homeopathic remedy before you have ever seen homeopathy at work and don't know what a remedy is, don't expect an accurate yes or no. On the other hand, if you have read several books on homeopathy and your healing issue is a simple one, ask your pendulum if a particular remedy is right for you. You will probably get good information. And in the health food store, where there are fifteen remedies displayed in several different potencies, the pendulum can be used to verify the remedy and help you pick which strength to buy.

The reason the pendulum works is that people only use five to ten percent of their brain capacity in a conscious way, and no one really knows why such a small portion of the human brain is active. But the other 90 percent has purpose, too. If you give a woman a newspaper and fifteen seconds reading time, she remembers the headlines and maybe another bit or two of information when you take it away. If you hypnotize that same woman, she remembers what the whole page said, because her brain picked up and stored the information on a subconscious level. A pendulum helps to access stored and only erratically used information.

Pendulum answers are also limited to Yes and No, and possibly to a Maybe or Don't Know made by the pendulum's hanging steadily or not registering. Therefore, how you phrase your questions becomes important. First of all, you can ask only for yes and no answers. Secondly, you can only ask for information already stored, and thirdly, it is necessary to phrase the questions without ambiguities or abstractions. For example, if you ask it "Will this flower remedy make me well?" you are not likely to get a meaningful answer. Better to ask, "Is this flower remedy positive for me?" or "Will this flower remedy help in my healing?" It takes a variety of things, inside and out, to make a woman well, and while the remedy may help, it alone is not likely to provide a 'cure.' The pendulum in this case could give a No, because it alone won't make you well, but would give clearer information if you asked, "Will it help?" The questions have to be very specific; they can't be too broad for the Yes or No to be meaningful.

For a fourth tip, keep your mind in a neutral emotional state while asking questions. Fifth, keep your body's energy circuit clear and uncrossed. Hold your arms and legs straight and not touching each other, feet firm on the floor, and avoid working around a lot of operating electrical appliances.[5] Be as specific as possible in the questions you ask, and state them as clearly as possible in the present tense. Like other skills, pendulums require use and practice, and the more you work with them, the more you learn when to trust their accuracy and when not to. Pendulums are not oracles. They will predict the future inaccurately. If your pendulum contains crystals or gemstones, reemember to clear its energies often.

There are several ways to use pendulums in healing, in choices and diagnosis. I use my pendulum this way in healthfood (or book, or gemstone) stores: I hold it over an item I consider buying and ask if it is positive for me. For example, I use it to see if a type of vitamin is useful for me, say vitamin C. Then I go to all the brands of vitamin C, swinging the pendulum over them, looking for a Yes over the best one for my needs, the right brand, amount, size, etc. Sometimes one brand will be a No and the next a Yes, both for vitamin C and the same number of milligrams. Vitamins are processed differently, so this is logical. Using vitamins at home, when a bottle is running out, I ask my pendulum, "Do I still need this?" or "Should I buy this again?" I also use the pendulum to determine dosage, "Should I take one of these a day? Two? Three? Should I take it with breakfast? Dinner?" Use this on a lot of other things besides vitamins to narrow down what you need, how much of it, when to use it. It takes some time to ask a series of simple questions, but the answers that way are accurate. Again, only ask the pendulum about things that your subconscious mind has information on.

When discussing different methods of healing, use the pendulum to choose which method is best, or ask it whether or not this particular healing system is positive for you at this time. Ask it to help you with almost any decision other than moral ones. The most accurate answers come when there is no bias one way or another in the choice. I use a pendulum to choose gemstones, vitamins, homeopathics (along with a lot of study), what herbs to put in a healing mix for myself or someone else. The pendulum works for others, as long as you have permission to gain the answers for them. I've asked it such questions as, "Should the dog go to the vet, or should I wait another day?"

In dietary issues or food allergies, ask the pendulum to help you find what item is the problem. In a long page of items, several columns, read the column first, then ask your pendulum, "Is there any food in this column that I'm allergic to?" If the pendulum says No, go on to the next column with the same question. If it's a Yes, run your finger along the items until the pendulum reacts. Use your receiving hand on the page and your sending hand to hold the pendulum.

Once I was undergoing great stress and my hair was falling out. A woman diagnosed me with muscle testing and put me on a number of vitamins. I felt better, but the hair didn't grow back. One day I asked my pendulum, just on a hunch, "Is this a food allergy?" and got a Yes. I went over everything I ate that might not be good for me and came up with a Yes on the chocolate ice cream I was eating almost every day after dinner. The pendulum said it was not ice cream, but chocolate that was the problem, and that I could eat it once in a while but not every day. I switched to a different flavor, breaking the chocolate allergy, and my hair began to grow back within a month. I had asked the pendulum when I'd see a difference and got the answer—a month. I also used the pendulum to help me choose herbs to encourage hair growth and internal cleansing. A chronic skin rash disappeared when I stopped eating chocolate. Food allergies can come from any food, including things good for you, but first suspect chocolate, dairy products, items containing refined flour, white sugar, and wheat.

In choosing gemstones for healing, use a pendulum to help decide what type of stone, and which specific ones you need right now. In a laying on of stones, use it to determine gemstone placements, such as where the geode goes. I use my pendulum to tell me when my stones need clearing, and whether I should use or not use a particular gemstone, or a particular healing method for a woman I'm working with.

A pendulum can be used to find which meridians are blocked and need acupressure or reflexology. A pendulum can also be used in polarity balancing to channel out blocked energy.[6] Here is how to do it. Holding your cleared pendulum in your sending hand, extend the index and middle finger of your other hand out toward another woman, about one to three inches away from her third eye. Slowly move those fingers (a plus and minus charge) back to her crown, down the back center of her head, and down her neck and spine, the line of the chakras, along her governing vessel meridian. If your pendulum swings a Yes, there is an excess of plus energy at that point, and a No means an excess of minus energy. Note the places for each.

Return to an excess plus point, holding the middle finger only (plus finger) of your receiving hand over it, and the pendulum in your other hand. The pendulum will swing a Yes until the excess is balanced. The energy can be neutralized by doing this while holding the pendulum tip over a bowl of water or a candle flame. For an excess minus spot, do the same thing, but use your index (minus) finger. If the pendulum changes directions, change fingers until the energy registers neutral. Long term issues take longer to balance than shorter ones. When all of the energy imbalances are righted, stop and brush off the woman's aura. Make sure to clear your pendulum, especially a crystal one, of the energies it has absorbed, and remember to ground yourself.

In a group pendulum healing from Anya Fields, using the above healing method, the woman with the pendulum finds the blocked meridian points. She puts her middle finger on a plus point, then another woman puts her middle finger on the knuckle of the first woman's finger. The next woman puts her middle finger on the second woman's knuckle, etc. All use the middle finger for a plus point or index finger for a minus one. When the first woman's pendulum changes direction, all of the women change fingers. Energy is balanced very quickly this way, with so many women participating.[7]

There can be rapid progress with this type of healing or slower, less perceptible healing. Sometimes the woman experiencing a healing of this type, or another type of women's healing, goes through what is called a healing crisis, in which she temporarily seems to get sicker. It can manifest as diarrhea, a cold, a headache, etc. Recovery from this is rapid, with the woman much better after than she was before the healing. There is usually an elimination of toxins involved in a healing crisis. Homeopathy calls this an aggravation, and considers it very positive, and it also occurs in reflexology.

Muscle testing works for the same reasons as the pendulum, using subconscious information translated through the meridian lines and ki of woman's body. Unlike the pendulum, which is used alone, muscle testing requires two women working together to use it. It gives the same yes and no answers as the pendulum does, working closely with the Goddess-within knowledge of what a woman needs for healing. It is a beginning of applied kinesiology, a process which corrects muscle weakness after finding the weakness through the testing.

The technique of muscle testing is derived again from the *Nei Jing* and from the ancient Chinese systems of acupuncture and the meridian flow of ki. Written material on Chinese healing goes back to 2500 BCE. Muscle testing as an outgrowth of Chinese healing has been developed in the west primarily by chiropractors using applied kinesiology. The developers include an osteopath, Dr. Frank Chapman; several chiropractors, Drs. Terrence Bennett, George Goodheart and John Thie, and a holistic psychiatrist, frustrated with the medical system, Dr. John Diamond.[8] Diamond was the one who popularized muscle testing for laywomen, making the process very simple. John Thie developed the Touch For Health system from it; both were students of George Goodheart. This is not to say that muscle testing or applied kinesiology are male medical fields. On the contrary, they came from early, probably matriarchal healing systems, and are practiced today by a large number of woman chiropractors and lay healers. The process of muscle testing can be particularly simple and available to women's healing.

Muscle testing is based on the concept that any stimulus added to the body, emotions, mind or spirit is either positive or negative for a woman's health. In pendulum work there is a neutral or Maybe, but in muscle testing there is only the Yes or No. A tested object—vitamin, herb, flower essence, homeopathic remedy, food, gemstone, etc.—either tests yes or no, positive or negative for the woman's well-being. The item being tested is held in the woman's receiving hand or in her mouth, touches her crown chakra or navel, or is even something she hears in a spoken statement. The woman's subconscious/emotional body gives the answers, through the code of the muscle test. By the muscle testing process, as with the pendulum, the woman's Goddess-within is brought to conscious translation.

To do a muscle testing, two women stand facing each other. The woman being tested raises either arm out straight to shoulder height. The woman testing her puts one hand on the woman's opposite shoulder to steady her, then places her other hand behind the flexed wrist of the woman being tested's outstretched arm. She tells the woman to 'hold' or 'resist,' then presses down slowly on the woman's arm above her wrist. The arm will probably lock and remain straight out, and the tester stops pressing. The lock is a Yes and says that the woman's arm is strong. No stimulus interferes at this point.

Now try it again, this time putting a lump of white sugar in the woman's receiving hand. When the tester says 'hold' and presses down on the woman's outstretched wrist, her arm goes down. It does not lock, and the woman is unable to resist the tester's pressure. This is a No, and says that the sugar is not positive for the woman's well-being. A stimulus that is positive for her and strengthens her gets a Yes, her arm remains extended. A stimulus that is negative for her, that weakens her, gives a No, and her arm goes down.[9] Try other other negative stimuli such as a negative statement, a plastic baggie placed on her crown chakra, a piece of white bread in her hand or mouth, a junk food cupcake, an aspirin or an over-the-counter drug, a food she is allergic to, or have her look at a fluorescent light. Then test her arm again without the negative stimulus. Try positive stimuli: a good multiple vitamin, a piece of whole wheat bread, a live flower in her hand (if she is not allergic to them), a positive affirmation, the sound of a song she likes, and watch the difference. Her arm locks and remains extended, her body says Yes.

This is the basic process of a simple muscle testing. There are some added instructions and tips for best results, though most of these are more optimal than necessary. Do testing in a neutral-colored room, and particularly in a room without fluorescent lighting. Wear neutral-colored clothing to test or be tested in, and remove all metal from your body—jewelry, metal watchbands, keys from pockets, belt buckles, etc. For best results clothes should not have metal zippers. Even remove eyeglasses with metal frames or trims. Keep the room quiet, without noise or music. These are optimal.

For necessary tips, neither woman should have food in her mouth or hands at the time of the testing, unless that food is being tested. This goes for vitamins or other items, as well. The woman being tested holds her body straight and faces straight ahead, finding a neutral spot on the wall to fix her eyes on. The woman doing the testing uses her palm to press behind the other woman's outstretched wrist. The tester presses down on the woman's arm, to feel its baseline strength, before adding an item to be tested. She says 'hold' or 'resist' before pressing.[10]

Do the pressing and releasing slowly and without force. The object is to see if the woman's arm will lock or fall, and it takes very little pressure for one or the other to happen, particularly if the tester has her hand in the right place, just behind the woman's flexed wrist. Too much pressure creates muscle strain and, in an experience of my own, pain in back and neck the next day. In that negative experience, my arm above the wrist was bruised black and blue after the testing. This is totally unnecessary and not to be tolerated. (I might add that this and the reflexology experience with the fingernails, both happened with male 'healers.' Women have more sense than to do these things.) The point is that force is not useful or necessary in muscle testing. If the answer is No, the woman's arm drops without much pressure. Practice this a few times to learn how much pressure to use. If even gentle testing causes a woman pain, go to the pendulum instead, or use a surrogate (see below) who may be less sensitive.

Use muscle testing as described so far for any number of healing choices. To ask if a particular vitamin, homeopathic remedy, herb or flower essence is helpful for a woman, place the item in her hand or under her tongue. If the item is strengthening to her meridian system, to the flow of ki and well-being through her body, her arm registers a Yes. If she gets a No with a particular vitamin, she might try the test again with a different brand or size of the same type.

To determine dosage amount, and how many a day, put varying amounts in her hand for testing and pick the one that gives the Yes. For time of day, the tester says aloud, "with dinner" or "with breakfast" when she presses the woman's arm. Use muscle testing to determine if a particular gemstone is a strengthener for the woman, if she is allergic to a food, if she should include more or less of a food in her diet, if she should continue or stop using a particular healing method or item. A woman chiropractor used muscle testing to determine if my new eyeglasses were right for me, since they weren't comfortable yet. She tested nonverbally, and I was not aware of her question to influence the response. The glasses were incorrect, and a return to the optometrist verified it.

Occasionally a woman shows responses in testing that seem

illogical. On first testing, her arm falls immediately with no stimulus there to weaken it. Something known to be positive for her gets a No, or a lump of sugar in her hand gets a Yes. The woman is often left-handed, and often says that she receives energy from her right (rather than her left) hand. She may be ambidextrous or dyslexic. If all or some of these things seem to be happening, the woman's energy circuits may be switched. This can be something particular to her or can be caused by the interference of such things as fluorescent lights in the testing room. Changing the energy circuit benefits her by immediately helping her resist the lights, and more important by helping her well-being. Switching it makes muscle testing possible, but the switching may be only temporary.

To uncross the energy flows and make the correction, use acupressure points, placing pressure on the designated meridians until the blockage releases. Brisk rubbing is usually enough. One set of points is on the kidney meridian, on both sides of her collarbone at the edges of the hollow of her throat. Another point is on her conception vessel at her navel, and again about an inch below to the right of her navel. Further points, less important for this situation, are on the tops of the woman's feet, about an inch back from the lowest bones of her toes. Between each top-of-foot bone there is a meridian point, four of them in a row across, and one more on the side of her foot on the big toe side.[11]

For the points at her navel, use two fingers together to press in deeply below the flesh and fat layer, or massage deeply. This is the most used point for unswitching. For the clavicle points, use thumb and first finger to press both sides. After releasing the meridian points, try testing again. It can take more than one try for the circuits to uncross. Priscilla Kapel suggests that persistent cross-switching can indicate nutritional imbalances or metal toxicities. A woman who needs to be unswitched once will need to be again for each muscle testing session. If the interference is from the environment, taking her outdoors for testing may be enough.

If the woman being tested is unable to participate actively, or if it is painful to her to have the tester press on her arm, she can still be tested by using a surrogate. This is also helpful when working with animals or small children. Muscle testing with a surrogate requires a third woman, who places her left hand on the woman being tested, while the tester presses on the surrogate's outstretched other arm for the response. Her contact with the first woman is important, as by touching her she channels the woman's energy pattern. If the woman is being tested for an herb, let's say, the herb is placed in the woman's hand, and then the surrogate

Switching Corrections

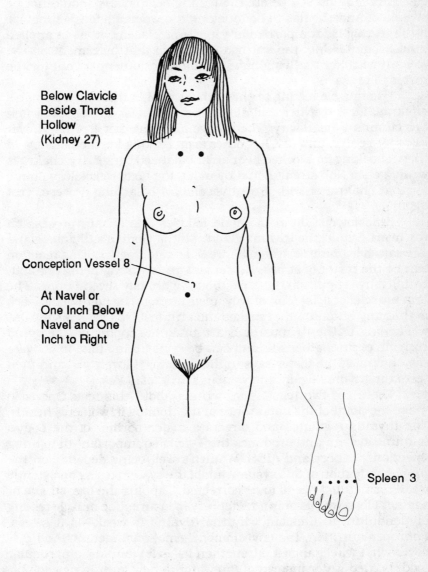

Below Clavicle
Beside Throat
Hollow
(Kidney 27)

Conception Vessel 8

At Navel or
One Inch Below
Navel and One
Inch to Right

Spleen 3

touches the woman. If the herb is strengthening for the woman, the surrogate's arm resists the tester's pressure. The surrogate should test strong by herself before the testing begins, she should not be switched, and she has to be touching the woman she is acting for. If the testing is for a particular muscle or placement, as in applied kinesiology testing, the surrogate touches that placement on the woman with her receiving hand, holding her other arm out for the tester to press.[12]

Use muscle testing to check the flow of ki through a woman's chakras. First test her arm alone; it should test strong. Unswitch her circuits if necessary. Then, have her place her free hand over her root center, and test her other arm. Do this for each chakra in turn, checking for blocked ki or an imbalanced center. If a chakra is weak (gets a No), strengthen it by using the body reflexology points for that chakra, or with any other chakra balancing process. Test again.

Kinesiologist John Diamond focuses this chakra process on the heart center, the thymus gland.[13] If the woman's thymus gland is weak, her immune system is weak or underactive. This reaction can be the result of stress. He demonstrates strengthening or activating it by tapping on the breastbone vigorously several times. The arm muscle, at least temporarily, tests strong. The point of his work is that any stimulus that makes the arm test No (weakens) is also weakening to the thymus or heart chakra. Tapping on the gland corrects or strengthens it, and can be done at any time to activate the chakra. If the tester says to the woman, "I love you," and then tests the thymus again, the woman's arm tests Yes.

There are two reasons for writing about this test. One is to make the point of the importance of the thymus in women's health. The thymus regulates and directs a major portion of the body's immune system and produces the T-cells so important in fighting infections, cancer and AIDS. Women's well-being depends on the proper activation of this system, and if the system tests consistently weak, something needs to be corrected. Tapping the breastbone or saying "I love you" is only a temporary measure. Use muscle testing or pendulum to find out why the thymus is weak—is it stress, improper nutrition, the environment, emotional factors? And discover what will change it, strengthen it—is it vitamins, a particular food, bottled water instead of tap water, a new lover, a new job?

The other reason is that it's a simple, very simple, description of an applied kinesiology healing. The process of applied kinesiology is to test an organ or muscle, and if it is weak, to do a movement or polarity that will strengthen it. The theory behind this is that each major muscle, like each meridian, is connected to an organ, and if the muscle tests weak (No), the organ is probably deficient in ki.[14] While muscle testing uses only the arm, the middle deltoid muscle, as an indicator, applied kinesiology uses over a hundred muscle points on the body in a variety of body positions. The woman experiencing this testing is usually lying on a massage or chiropractic table, and the practitioner manipulates her positions and tells her how and when to hold while she tests. If a muscle tests weak, the practitioner uses polarity, acupressure placements, or chiropractic adjusting to correct it. If her correction is successful, the muscle tests Yes on a re-test.

Applied kinesiology is very complicated and requires a thorough knowledge of physiology and of the muscles of the body. In Chinese healing, the requirement for this work was knowledge of the meridian system, with dozens of points on each of fourteen or twenty meridian channels. Most applied kinesiology today in the west is done by chiropractors, and it's an interesting and wonderful thing to experience. Instead of the force and twisting that many chiropractors use, applied kinesiology chiropractic is very gentle, balancing one energy point against another so that bones out of place move into position seemingly by themselves. Obviously, the process is too complicated for a book chapter, but muscle testing and using it to balance the chakras or test stimuli is a start. The Touch For Health process taught in various parts of the country is applied kinesiology, and recommended for women who are interested. However, it is very expensive.

Some information is given here on doing corrections for a muscle that tests weak or for a pain area. The corrections are basically acupressure and follow the meridian lines. To use the examples, locate the points it says to massage, test them for weak or strong by muscle testing and, if weak, massage or use pressure to release them. After massaging the meridian points indicated, test the placement again. To test a position, hold your receiving hand over the spot and your other arm out for the tester to press. The information gives some causes and a series of herbs, vitamins and foods for healing each dis-ease. Test each suggested item with muscle testing, say the word aloud if no sample is available, to see which suggestions are strengthening to the individual. Using an affirmation with each healing process and correction may be useful. Find them in Louise Hay's *You Can Heal Your Life*, (Santa Monica, CA, Hay House, 1984), or in any other source you choose. "I am strong, healthy and loved," is an example.

The muscle testing placements, massage positions, and herb

or vitamin suggestions for each dis-ease that follows are from Biokinesiology Institute, *Muscle Testing: Your Way to Health*, (Shady Cove, OR, Biokinesiology Institute, 1982). I disagree strongly with this book's patriarchal, god-righteous attitude, but it is the only simple material currently available to my knowledge on applied kinesiology-type lay healing. This is a field where information for the laywoman is sorely needed, and a field of great potential in women's healing. Most applied kinesiologists are woman chiropractors— won't one of you write us a teaching book? The healings below take two women to do, the one being tested and receiving the meridian corrections, and the other to do the testing and the massage/ acupressure with her. The woman may wish to do the massage herself, where she can reach it.

For recurrent **headaches**, test the woman's upper back muscles along her spine between her shoulder blades. If they test weak, work the acupressure points moving upward from her shoulder blade level to the top of her back. (These are also used in the shiatsu sequence.) Test again. Suggested sources to test for are allergy to vitamin B-5 (pantothenic acid), tomatoes, coconut, cantaloupe. Suggested healing information is vitamin C-complex, mineral complex, honey, white willow bark or white willow leaves.[15] Test the woman's arm for a Yes or No on these and follow the information accordingly. If an allergy is the cause and testing locates it, eliminate the food from your diet; if a food, herb or vitamin could strengthen you, try it and see what happens.

When the headaches occur behind the eyes or are sinus headaches, test the muscles located on the front and sides of the neck, massaging them deeply but gently if they test No. Possible causes are allergy to polyvinylchloride or the foam of foam mattresses, or a tender nerve or cavity in the lower front first molar. Possible healing information includes vitamins A, B-complex, B-12, cell salts or potassium-iodide.[16] B-complex may be especially positive.

If the headaches are frontal, test the muscles running up the back of the neck beside the spinal column to the skull. Allergies to vitamins A, E or F are possible, as are allergies to soy products, sage, honey or pancreatin. For healing suggestions, test for iron, mineral complex, pancreatin, cell salts, B-complex, brewer's yeast and licorice herb.[17] If these muscles are tense, an acupressure Neck Release can work wonders. Work the points on the muscles running up the neck and test again.

For **hypoglycemia**, test a placement along the center inside arm, about three-quarters of the way to the elbow crease. If the placement tests weak, find the acupressure meridian point and release it. The point is deep, so press hard. Other points are on the center line of the body from navel to breastbone (massage them upward), and the back of the upper arm moving downward. Also up the back side of the neck and down the inside lower arm. Test again after releasing the points. Healing suggestions include: vitamin E-complex, B-12, F, kelp, lecithin, mineral complex, cell salts, aduki beans, chia seeds, and soy protein powder.[18] Pantothenic acid (B-5) is mentioned here as a possible allergy, but is also a major recommendation in hypoglycemia healing. I have rarely found women with significant vitamin allergies but occasionally find allergies to the bindings used in making the vitamin tablets. Test different brands.

In a muscle testing for **high blood pressure**, check the muscles at the coccyx, pressing between spine and hipbone, and also the muscles of the upper back to the middle of the neck, on both sides of the spine. If one of these placements tests No, reflex the acupressure points and test again. Healing suggestions include: vitamins B-6, B-12, E, F, kelp, lecithin, mineral complex, potassium, zinc, cayenne, ginger, honey, columbine, papaya seed, red clover and yucca.[19] Also recommended are dong quai herb and Kyolic (odorless garlic perles).

For **menstrual pain** or irregular cycles, as well as difficult menopause, test the pressure point located in the muscular pad running from wrist to the lower thumb. Work the tender reflexes, then test again. Check the reflexes for the thyroid, pituitary and pineal glands in the hand. Suggestions to test: E-complex, lecithin, PABA and zinc.[20] Also try dong quai and raspberry leaf.

In ovarian or uterine **cysts** or pain in these organs, test the meridian point on the tragus of the ear, the little flap in the center, working the reflex if it tests weak. Healing suggestions include vitamin B-6, E-complex, lecithin, mineral complex, pancreatin and yellow dock.[21] Also check red clover with violet leaf herbs. For **yeast infections**, check on the lower half of the upper leg, just above the knee on the outside. If it tests weak, look for an acupressure point about six inches above the knee. Release the point and muscle test again. Also work on adrenal and thyroid reflexes. Test for calcium and PABA as healing suggestions.[22] Check for Kyolic, dong quai and acidophilus also.

For **sore throats**, check muscle placements under the jaw on the sides and from the middle of the breastbone to the shoulder. Also massage the throat area in circles, the entire area, and check the thigh position above the knee used for ovarian healing. Check these points and, if one tests weak, release the meridian reflexes, then test again. Do massage on the throat gently, under the jaw deeply but gently. The jaw points especially can be very tender. Check for possible allergies to honey, figs or raisins. Healing suggestions to test for include lecithin, E-complex, mineral complex, maple syrup, PABA and calcium. For tonsillitis, check meridian points that move out at the waist from the spinal column to the lower ribs on both sides. Add vitamin B-12, zinc and cell salts to the healing test suggestions, and test for possible allergies to garlic, vitamin A, iron or B-6.[23] Garlic (Kyolic) is a major healer for chronic tonsilitis and sore throats, so check that one too. See what makes you stronger and what weaker. These are only the briefest of lay beginnings of applied kinesiology in women's healing.

The question of what vitamin(s) or mineral(s) you need can be complicated, but muscle testing on resonant points can help. Resonant points are places on the aura, meridian points that have been mapped in this case for vitamin placement. When these points are touched with one hand while the other arm is muscle tested, the point tests weak if the woman is deficient for that vitamin or mineral. Double check it by placing one of the tablets of that supplement in the woman's receiving hand or mouth and testing again. If the arm resists strongly, the supplement is positive and strengthens her.[24] Before beginning the testing, unswitch the meridians, using pressure on the ends of the clavicle on either side of the throat chakra or at the navel. A few moments brisk massage is enough for this.

To evaluate the vitamins she is already taking, have her bring them to the testing session. If a vitamin tests weak, but the nutritional reflex test shows that she needs that vitamin, it may be the brand or size that is wrong for her. Vitamins are made with coatings and bindings that may be the problem. If she shows weakness at a vitamin point that requires another vitamin to assimilate (calcium requires D, for example), test the co-vitamin, as that may be the deficiency.

The test point for vitamin B is on the tongue, so have the woman put her finger in her mouth for the testing. There are a whole complex of B vitamins, say each one aloud and test it separately, while the woman keeps her free finger on the B vitamin test reflex. The B vitamins include B-1, B-2, B-3, B-5, B-6, B-12, B-13, B-15 and B-17, plus biotin, choline, inositol, folic acid and PABA.[25] When one of these is needed, a full B-complex should also be used.

Nutritional Reflexes for Muscle Testing

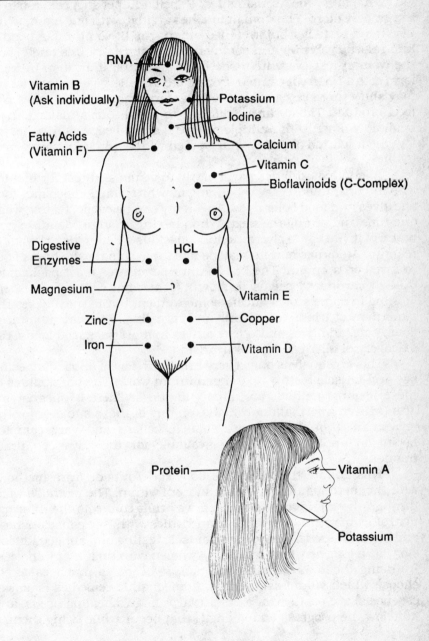

To test for food sensitivities, Priscilla Kapel suggests a trip to the grocery store. The woman touches an item with one hand, while her friend tests her outstretched other arm. (If you think a pendulum raises eyebrows and comments in a store, try this one!) Have the woman test every item she buys and eats. If an item in fresh form gets a No, try it canned, frozen, etc. An allergy to corn or wheat may show up more easily in the fresh form than when it's part of a food product. These can be difficult to avoid, but a major part of healing. Women with multiple sclerosis should especially be tested for wheat/gluten allergies, and women with asthma for corn sensitivity.

Allergy possibilities particularly to watch and test for include wheat, corn, milk, eggs, yeast, sugar, white flour, chocolate, food additives and food color dyes. An allergy can be cyclic, testing weak one time and strong the next. When testing an item, visualize how much of it you eat to give your subconscious a better idea of what to react to. An ounce of nuts may be fine for a woman who breaks out in hives on a cupful. The body's aura penetrates most packaging, though cardboard seems to slow it somewhat.[26] The fluorescent lighting in some stores affects some women, but in most cases the supermarket trip is interesting and revealing. With the amount of chemicals, additives and preservatives in most packaged foods, the discovery of allergies is not surprising.

This obviously is only a very brief overview of applied kinesiology and muscle testing and of pendulum work. The possibilities of these healing methods are almost limitless. There is surprisingly little written information available on any of these subjects for the laywoman, though there are some excellent and very complex books on applied kinesiology available for the advanced practitioner.

This chapter connects the bodywork/outside aura methods with the methods that influence ki from within. The methods work through the meridian system in a way that connects the information of woman's nonphysical aura bodies with her consciousness and physical levels. Pendulums, muscle testing and applied kinesiology go a long way toward helping women with their many choices. By using these as a diagnostic tool, it becomes much easier to choose which vitamin(s), herb(s), homeopathic remedies or flower essence(s) are positive for a particular woman's healing needs, and to follow the progress and changes that occur while using them.

NOTES

1. John Thie, DC, *Touch For Health*, (Marina del Rey, CA, DeVorss and Co. Publishers, 1979), p. 6. These numbers have much increased in the last ten years.

2. Diet means what you eat. I do not support the concept of reducing diets.

3. Greg Nielsen and Joseph Polansky, *Pendulum Power*, (Rochester, VT, Destiny Books, 1987), p. 16.

4. Anya Fields, *Dowsing Dykes*, (Milwaukee, WI, Crystal Revelations, 1982), pp. 14–15.

5. Greg Nielsen and Joseph Polansky, *Pendulum Power*, pp. 38–41.

6. This sequence is from Anya Fields, *Dowsing Dykes*, pp. 27–29. Also in Nett Hart and Lee Lanning, *Awakening*, (Minneapolis, Word Weavers, 1987), p. 130.

7. *Ibid.*, p. 29.

8. Priscilla Kapel, *The Body Says Yes*, (San Diego, CA, ACS Publications, 1981), pp. 3–4.

9. John Diamond, MD, *Your Body Doesn't Lie*, (New York, Warner Books, 1979), pp. 7–10.

10. Biokinesiology Institute, *Muscle Testing: Your Way to Health*, (Shady Cove, OR, Biokinesiology Institute, 1982), pp. 9–10.

11. Priscilla Kapel, *The Body Says Yes*, pp. 47–48.

12. *Ibid.*, pp. 53–56.

13. John Diamond, MD, *Your Body Doesn't Lie*, p. 42 ff.

14. *Ibid.*, p. 32.

15. Biokinesiology Institute, *Muscle Testing: Your Way to Health*, p. 49.

16. *Ibid.*, pp. 50 and 55.

17. *Ibid.*, pp. 51–52.

18. *Ibid.*, pp. 63–65.

19. *Ibid.*, pp. 32–33.

20. *Ibid.*, p. 72.

21. *Ibid.*, p. 75.

22. *Ibid.*, p. 94.

23. *Ibid.*, pp. 88–89 and 92.

24. Priscilla Kapel, *The Body Says Yes*, pp. 42–47.

25. *Ibid.*, pp. 45–46.

26. *Ibid.*, pp. 47–48.

Chapter Seven

───────○───────

Vitamins and Minerals

Vitamins are one of the latest known of healing methods and possibly the most commercialized and most controversial. They were recognized as being essential for health in 1906 and isolated for the first time in 1915 when a fat soluble food element was identified and extracted from butter, egg yolks and fish liver, and a water soluble one was extracted from wheat bran. In 1920, the fat soluble substance was labeled 'vitamin A' and the water soluble one 'vitamin B' simply to distinguish between the two. It was 1956 before the rest of the B-complex of vitamins was identified and numbers were given to them, B-1, B-2, etc. As other types of vitamins were discovered, they continued the alphabet for vitamins C, D, E, F, K, P and U.[1]

The substances were chemical mysteries until the structure of vitamin A was first understood in 1933. Vitamins were identified as the elements that prevented various dis-eases, but it was not known what these elements were. Vitamin C was known as the anti-scurvy factor, vitamin B-complex, the anti-beriberi substance, and vitamin D the anti-rickets element. It was known that the substances were nutritional after 1907 (scientists were looking for germs for these dis-eases before that), but because of the minute quantities involved and the difficulty in isolating them, their natures went unexamined for a long time. After 1933, the chemical structure of vitamin A was recognized, and in 1947 the vitamin was synthesized for the first time.[2] Since then, almost all vitamins have been synthesized, and that chemical process has been the basis for the vitamin/healthfood industry and the wide availability of vitamins and minerals. Minerals, which are of increasing importance, came later.

Even today, there is not much known about vitamins. Some

substances listed as vitamins may not be vitamins at all (PABA, inositol, the vitamin P bioflavinoids, pangamic acid/B-15, vitamin B-13, and coenzyme Q),[3] while others have sparked major controversies over what they are and can do (vitamin B-17/laetrile as a help for cancer, vitamin U for ulcers). Probably there are vitamins yet to be discovered. It is generally conceded that the lack of research and serious investigation has been caused by interference from the FDA (the Federal Food and Drug Administration) in this country, with the highly profitable and profiteering drug and food processing industries behind it.

The FDA's job is to prevent harm or misrepresentation in the composition, labeling and advertising of foods and drugs sold for human consumption. Since vitamins are not drugs, but occur naturally in the anatomy of all living things, the FDA's harassment is repressive and unfounded. Vitamins do great good and no harm, and the loud claims of toxicities are highly overblown. Only three vitamins contain overdose risks, vitamins A, D and K. Vitamin K is used for special needs and is available only by prescription; overdose effects of vitamins A or D are highly exaggerated—if they are overdosed the effects disappear as soon as the vitamins are stopped. With all the other vitamins, including fat soluble vitamin E, the excess is released from the body harmlessly by elimination. Mineral toxicities are rare.

Vitamins and minerals are natural substances (as are herbs), and as such they cannot be patented. The megalithic (and none too honest) drug industry controls the health market with patented pharmaceuticals that can be sold at inflated prices, whereas it cannot patent or control vitamins. The food processing industry has de-nutritionalized, de-vitaminized and over-chemicalized foods to the point where little nutrition is left in them. The industry does not want it known that vitamins are necessary for full nutrition and health. It's in both industries' interests to have vitamins off the market or under their control (listed as drugs to be monopolized by their own corporations), and this is where FDA pressure on the vitamin and healthfood industry originates.

The rigorous repression of vitamins that began in the 1960s was a red herring to deflect popular interest from more serious health issues, issues the FDA *should* have been controlling but wasn't. The 1960s saw the first major increases in food additives, chemical preservatives and colorings in foods and hormones in meats. The epidemic of processed foods and fast foods with little or no nutrition was growing by leaps and bounds, and rumblings of drug side effects and disasters began to be heard.

Many critics accused the FDA of using the vitamin issue as a smokescreen to avoid dealing with more serious matters, such as drug safety and the misleading packaging of foods. To investigate these other, more important issues would mean stepping on too many big business toes, said the critics, so the FDA used the vitamin issue (which it knew would attract much attention) to present the image of a vigorous regulating agency devoted to public welfare.[4]

Some of these issues were the increasing use of hormone therapies on women. By 1960, the FDA knew that hormones in pregnancy would cause birth defects, and early warnings that the pill caused phlebitis were beginning by 1962. Deaths were reported with the IUD by 1965, and estrogen replacement therapies began in the 1960s, for the most part untested, that later proved to be highly carcinogenic.[5] The thalidomide birth defect tragedy and the vaginal cancers in daughters of women who used DES to prevent miscarriage became known later. These and the increase in untested or half-tested (or corporation-tested) drugs on the market with their later discovered side effects and dangers were among the issues the FDA was not investigating when it chose to attack vitamins. Every woman should list Barbara and Gideon Seaman's *Women and the Crisis in Sex Hormones*, (New York, Rawson Associates, 1977) as required reading about these deadly drug scams.

With all of this going on, the Food and Drug Administration began its war on vitamins in the 1960s. First they set legal Minimum Daily Requirements (MDRs) that were not to be exceeded for vitamin intake, based on very little nutritional research. They set a number of limitations on amounts, sales and information dissemination for vitamin and mineral supplements that continue today. In 1968, they exchanged the MDRs to Recommended Daily Allowances (RDAs), and to the Recommended Dietary Allowances in 1974.[6] Each scale of recommendations lowered the legal amounts for each vitamin, and the limits are now so low as to be inconsequential. European standards followed the FDA's. The result of this is that a processed food manufacturer can advertise that it contains the Recommended Dietary Allowance of, say B-complex, when it does not in any way contain the daily amount needed for health. It can advertise 50 percent of the daily requirement for calcium, vitamin D or whatever, and include very little nutrition while claiming how nutritional it is. The manufacturer also uses synthetic vitamins as supplements which are next to worthless.

The government figures are based on how much of a vitamin or mineral it takes to prevent a deficiency dis-ease—as in how much vitamin C it takes to prevent scurvy—rather than on what is needed for optimal good health. The FDA continues to claim that any necessary vitamins are obtained from food but continues to promote the nutritional deterioration of foods in a variety of ways. There is no recognition of individual dietary or health needs. Laws on labeling prevent a vitamin or mineral bottle from listing what the supplement is *for*, other than saying that it's a dietary supplement. In 1974, along with the Recommended Dietary Allowances, the government proposed to list as a drug and therefore legally control any vitamin that contained more than 150 percent of its RDA amount. The bill was defeated, but rumblings of new attacks on vitamins and the healthfood industry are heard every few years. The limitations and low legal amounts set by the FDA for most vitamins are only a fraction of real nutritional needs.

As usual, women lose out to the patriarchal establishment, and a totally safe and beneficial healing method is misrepresented. Radio blurbs equate vitamins with quacks and say that no one who eats properly needs them.

From years of reading and experience, I feel that every woman needs vitamins. The very sections of big business that work to repress the vitamin industry are the reasons that vitamins are so needed as supplements to the best nutrition women can find today. The propaganda from the FDA and the mislabeling of foods is particularly tragic because it takes this information away from less informed people who may need vitamins the most and lulls them into believing that their nutritionless processed foods contain all they need. The nonwhite poor, the handicapped and elders, women and children are receiving misinformation that negatively effects their health. And since vitamins are not drugs by FDA standards or foods by the US Department of Agriculture definition, they are not paid for by Medicaid, Medicare or food stamps. Since most of the poor are women, it is women and children who are being nutritionally deprived.

The patriarchy's tamperings with Goddess Earth make vitamin supplementation necessary. In the days of the matriarchies, and for thousands of years after, foods were grown organically—that is, without chemical fertilizers or insecticides. Sweets were derived from honey, not white cane sugar, and grains were whole grains, not white flour or white rice products. Cancer, heart disease, high blood pressure, AIDS, multiple sclerosis, and most of the other degenerative dis-eases that are killing women today were unheard of or rare in the 1920s and later. Foods grown in good soil, watered with clean water, and not poisoned with chemicals proba-

THE FDA IS TRYING TO PUT YOU OUT OF BUSINESS.

FDA officials have started a new harrassment campaign against health-food stores and have announced that they are going to close all health-food stores in the country, one at a time.

The FDA says that by calling your store a health-food store, you are making claims for your products, and that they are therefore drugs, and that you are therefore illegally selling drugs.

Congress has passed no law giving the FDA this power. What they are doing is illegal, and they have already started. They came to my store last week with a search warrant and put embargo tags on half a ton of health foods, with a notice that anyone moving same will be arrested.

My store didn't even have a sign that said "Health Food Store" and had never been advertised as a health-food store, but that didn't matter to the FDA.

I'm sure I could win in court, but legal fees would be in excess of $50,000, in addition to the loss of the products embargoed (they will be too old to sell by the time the embargo is lifted), plus two or three years out of business.

I am not as young as some of you, and this forces me to retire from the health-food business. I will be devoting more time to investigating the FDA. The FDA invaders who raided my store had orders straight from Washington, and they have orders from Washington to raid your store, also.

You may be next.

The time to stop them is before they invade your store, embargo your goods and close your doors. The time to do something is now. What can you do?

Write to your congressperson and tell him or her that you want a congressional investigation of the FDA.

It worked when we (the Committee for Honesty in Government) asked Congress to investigate the U.S. Attorney General (John Mitchell, at the time). They responded by putting him behind bars. At that time, our funds were meager, and our campaign was very small. Several congressmen said that they received only two or three letters, but that those letters were very convincing, and swayed their votes in favor of an investigation.

This time, we have a much broader campaign. Our funds are substantial, and our organization is much larger. With a little help from each health-food store, we can soon expect Congress to start its investigation, and we have a mountain of evidence to submit to the congressional investigating committee.

We are not giving an address because we are not asking for donations. We have enough money; we have enough volunteers. All we ask you to do is to give out the enclosed letters, have more printed, and write your congressman. The business you save may be your own.

Flyer found in a health food store in September, 1987.

bly still contain all the vitamins and minerals women need, if we could find them. The trouble is that we can't. The patriarchy's policy of conquer and dominate has left us with universally polluted and chemicalized water, air and soil. White flour and white sugar, the staple American diet, is absolutely and totally without nutritional value. Americans consume an average of a hundred pounds of sugar per person per year.[7] American aid to 'underdeveloped' countries include such foods that are no one's answer to world hunger.

There are a number of reasons why women cannot get full nutrition from modern food, even women who avoid refined products and fast foods, choosing instead raw vegetables, whole grains and healthier diets.

1. Soil depletion from abuse and overcropping is becoming the norm. Food grown on such soils, however chemically fertilized, is nutritionally poor. Chemical fertilizers produce bigger crops, but not nutritionally better ones.

2. Toxic insecticides and chemical fertilizers are used universally in agriculture today. They leave residues on food and in the soil and destroy beneficial organisms to further harm the earth, creating a vicious cycle of needing more and more chemicals for the same crop results.

3. Much produce is picked and shipped before ripe; ripening on the vine or tree is essential to full vegetable or fruit nutrition.

4. The use in food of dyes, waxes, detergents, emulsifiers, bleaches, etc. is pervasive. I get quite disturbed when my cucumbers are waxed too slippery to pick up and leave green stains on the sink top. Undyed oranges are not orange, but yellow-green, and most women have never seen them that way.

5. White sugar is as much as one fourth of the American diet, and is totally nutrition-free.

6. Chemical additives, preservatives, dyes and artificial ingredients which may cause harm and have no nutritional value, are used indiscriminately. Many of these are known to be toxic, but the FDA moves slowly or not at all to test and regulate them. Over 1200 FDA approved items have never been tested for safety. Remember the past publicity over Red Dye Number Two, saccharine and cyclamates?[8] If you can't pronounce an item on the box, you probably shouldn't eat it.

7. The increasing pollution by toxic wastes, chemical and industrial wastes and spills into the water supply, air and soil, help to pollute food crops. Also the carbon monoxide and lead levels from automobiles, buses, trucks and airplanes are deadly. Regulation of

big business to stop this pollution is too limited to be significant.

8. Radioactivity and radioactive wastes from nuclear testing, nuclear accidents and nuclear power plants reach the soil and the food grown on it.

9. The proposed irradiation of foods, including spices, herbs, grains, fruits and vegetables, meats, poultry, milk products, fish and nuts—virtually everything—is now beginning. Losses of twenty to eighty percent are listed for vitamins A, B-complex, C, E, F and K in these products. FDA rulings propose to lift the requirement that irradiated items be labeled. The whole unsavory project seems to be the baby of the nuclear and food processing industries.[9]

10. The pervasiveness of fast food restaurants and their heavy marketing policies do not help American nutrition. What they serve is filling but is not food.

There are differences in individual needs for vitamins and minerals. High stress depletes many vitamins rapidly in the body, particularly vitamin C. Pregnancy, lactation, menstruation and menopause increase or change a woman's vitamin and mineral needs. Digestive disturbances deplete vitamins in the body rapidly, as most vitamins are absorbed from the intestines. Fevers also deplete vitamins rapidly. Use of antibiotics destroys many vitamins, as do drugs and medications of all types, even simple things like antacids. Alcohol, caffeine and cigarettes destroy the body's vitamins and vitamin balance as well. A woman who is a vegetarian needs more of the B-complex vitamins than a woman who is a meat-eater, and highly active women have different nutritional needs than more sedentary ones. Women with any dis-ease or illness have highly individualized vitamin needs, different from when they are in top health. Once a woman is deficient in a vitamin or mineral, it takes a far larger amount than the actual deficiency to make up for it, as much as ten to fifty times more daily.[10]

From even this brief overview, it is clear that women need to know about vitamins and minerals. The issue is not as simple as going to the grocery store and buying a bottle of something, anything. A supermarket daily vitamin that claims it's all you need by the standards of the RDAs is next to worthless. A brief description of each vitamin follows, with some tips on how to use it. I recommend for anyone using vitamin supplements first to get a *good* (not cheap, but good) multiple vitamin from a quality manufacturer that contains both vitamins and minerals in a solid balance. My own choice is Sunrider's Meta-Balance 44 or Schiff's Single Day, but there are other good ones on the market. I use the multiple vitamin twice a day with meals. Look for vitamins that are

Vitamins and Minerals

Vitamin/ Mineral	RDA Adult Amount	Recommended for Women of Average Weight		
		Age 22–25	Age 36–60	Over 60
A	5000 IU	20,000 IU	20,000 IU	20,000–30,000
D	400 IU	800 IU	800 IU	800–1200
E	30 IU	200–400 IU	400–1200 IU	800–1200
C	60 Mg	1000–5000 Mg	1000-5000 Mg	1000–5000
B-1 (Thiamine)	1.5 Mg	100–200 Mg	150–300 Mg	200–300
B-2 (Riboflavin)	1.7 Mg	50–100 Mg	100–300 Mg	150–300
B-3 (Niacin)	20 Mg	200–1000 Mg	200–1000 Mg	400–2000
B-5 (Pantothenic Acid)	10 Mg	100–200 Mg	100–200 Mg	100–200
B-6 (Pyridoxine)	2 Mg	200–600 Mg	300–800 Mg	100–600
B-12 (Cyano-cobalamine)	6 Mcg	25–75 Mcg	25–75 Mcg	25–75
Biotin	0.3 Mg	0.3–0.6 Mg	0.3–0.6 Mg	0.3–0.6
Choline		250–1000 Mg	250–1000 Mg	250–1000
Folic Acid (B-9)	0.4 Mg	2–5 Mg	2–5 Mg	2–5
Inositol		500 Mg	500–1000 Mg	1000
PABA		100 Mg	100 Mg	200
F (EFA-Essential Fatty Acids)		10–20 Gm	10–20 Gm	10–20
Calcium	0.6 Gm	1–2 Gm		
Phosphorus	0.5 Gm	1–2 Gm		
Iodine	45 Mcg	150–300 Mcg		
Iron	15 Mg	20–60 Mg		
Magnesium	70 Mg	400–800 Mg		
Copper	0.6 Mg	2–4 Mg		
Zinc	5 Mg	15–30 Mg		

natural, not synthetic, and that are sugar free, wheat free, dye free and yeast free.

The reason for the multiple vitamin is that many vitamins and minerals require balancing with other vitamins and minerals in order to work. For example, calcium requires vitamin D, and the B-complex vitamins require each other. A good multiple vitamin is balanced. If you need additional individual vitamins, follow these tips. When taking vitamin C, look for one that contains the bioflavinoids (vitamin P, or C-complex), and since C washes out of the body quickly in the urine, use time-release C. Vitamin E contains a series of tocopherols, and is sometimes sold as E-complex. Buy natural E for effectiveness, marked d-alpha-tocopherols, rather than synthetic E marked dl-alpha-tocopherols. E is one of the few vitamins I recommend getting a quality brand for—E can become rancid if it sits around or is processed poorly. Other than E, a cheaper brand is fine if you know what you are buying and have no allergies to the fillers.

Vitamins A and D usually come together. There is a dry form that makes overdosing highly unlikely. Vitamin E also comes in dry form. If you are iron deficient, try a B-complex (B-complex-50, or even 100) before starting with iron supplements that are hard to take and cause constipation. Vitamin B-12, cyanocobalamine, is the transporting mechanism for the body's iron, and the deficiency may be there instead of in iron itself. Iron and calcium are the two most frequent vitamin deficiencies for women.[11] You may be calcium deficient if you have menstrual cramps, premenstrual syndrome (PMS) or muscle spasms in your legs at night. Calcium is vitamin D dependent and should also be used with half as much magnesium for best results. Women with magnesium deficiencies also crave chocolate before their periods.

Here is a survey of vitamins and minerals from A to Z, based on experience and the following books: Velma Keith and Monteen Gordon, *The How To Herb Book*, (Pleasant Grove, UT, Mayfield Publishing Co, 1984), Harold Rosenberg, *The Book of Vitamin Therapy* (New York, Berkeley Books, 1974), and Earl Mindell's *Vitamin Bible*, (New York, Warner Books, 1985). *The How To Herb Book* is the most important and most recommended of these for both vitamins and herbs.

Vitamin A, a fat soluble vitamin (along with D, E and K), was the first vitamin to be identified and synthesized. A is an antioxidant, which means that it protects cells from uncontrolled oxidations. Pollutants are oxidants, and vitamin A is a protection from pollutants. In vegetables, the vitamin comes from beta carotene (and can be bought in that form as pro-vitamin A), the factor that the body changes to vitamin A in the assimilation process. Beta carotene is water soluble and without overdose risk, but some women with A deficiencies are not able to assimilate it. While vitamin A is one of the vitamins that can be overdosed, women are more likely to have too little rather than too much. Vitamin E, protein, choline, essential fatty acids (vitamin F) and zinc are needed for assimilation of vitamin A, and it is recommended that you take zinc when you are using it.

Deficiency symptoms of vitamin A include eye disorders, itching eyes and eye strain, rough skin, dry hair, recurrent infections, appetite and weight loss, impaired sense of smell and night blindness. It helps in such dis-eases as acne, boils, emphysema, hyperthyroidism, respiratory infections, allergies and hay fever, and is an anti-cancer agent. Vitamin A builds strong bones, promotes children's growth, extends life, aids in protein digestion, helps the eyes, skin, hair, teeth and gums, and is a protection against environmental pollution. Adults have taken as much as 100,000 IU a day of vitamin A, and infants 18,000 IU a day for many months without toxicities. Women who take the pill need *less* vitamin A, and women who take more than 400 IU of vitamin E daily need more than the suggested[12] minimum 10,000 IU of A per day.

Vitamin D is also fat soluble, and often comes with vitamin A supplements. D is produced on the skin when the body is exposed to the sun and sunstroke may be triggered by an excess of this vitamin. Since many women see sun only for four days a year at the Michigan Women's Music Festival, and since the sun's rays in cities are screened by pollution and made toxic by the destruction of the ozone layer, vitamin D is absolutely necessary. Natural vitamin D is nontoxic in doses up to 100,000–150,OOO IU daily over a long period (recommended amounts are about 800 IU per day) but may be more toxic with synthetic than natural forms of it. Moslem women forced to remain fully covered outdoors develop osteoporosis and bone dis-eases readily, as do nuns in long habits and women who work at night. Vitamin D and calcium deficiencies are implicated in the high rates of osteoporosis among elder women. Black women in northern climates are also more susceptible than white women to deficiencies. Smog and mineral oil destroy vitamin D in the body.

Therapy with vitamin D has proved positive for women who are epileptics. Other indications are in bone, tooth or skin dis-eases and for arthritis, myopia or conjunctivitis and to prevent colds (with A and C). Vitamin D helps women's bodies absorb calcium and phosphorus; it works best with these and with vitamins A and C.

Vitamin E is a miracle vitamin that aids and promotes any form of healing and regeneration in women's bodies. Though a fat soluble vitamin, it is stored in the body only for a short time and then released, and it is therefore nontoxic in any amount. I have taken as much as 1600 IU a day for months with good results; the suggested amount is about 400 IU a day (RDA is 30 IU). Before elective surgery, take 1600 IU a day of E for about two weeks, and take it for two to four weeks after to aid healing. Vitamin E requires manganese in the body to be effective and selenium increases its potency and effects. Like vitamin D, mineral oil and smog destroy this vitamin, and also saturated fats. Do not take vitamin E within eight hours of an inorganic iron supplement as the E will be destroyed. If you have chlorinated drinking water, you need more vitamin E.

E is positive for fertility, and is known as the burn vitamin. It is the best skin remedy available. Poke a hole in a vitamin E capsule with a needle and use the contents externally. I have had persistent, itching rashes disappear in an hour with it. It is an antioxidant that protects women's bodies against pollution and secondary cigarette smoke, and it retards aging. Use it with vitamin A. Vitamin E helps to prevent miscarriages, reduces scars, helps leg cramps (also try calcium with magnesium), and reduces high blood pressure and heart dis-ease. Increased E is recommended for pregnant or nursing women, women on the pill or estrogen, and is highly recommended in menopause to decrease hot flashes. Vitamin E is a major anti-cancer agent, particularly against breast cancers.

Women with high blood pressure, arteriosclerosis and heart dis-ease find their best ally in vitamin E. For these dis-eases, begin with very small amounts daily and work up gradually, increasing each month from 90 IU. Vitamin E increases blood circulation and oxygen levels and dissolves blood clots. The vitamin's detergent action can temporarily increase cholesterol readings as the deposits are moved from the heart and arteries, so do it slowly. For this reason blood pressure can temporarily increase and then will greatly decrease. Women with these dis-eases should start slowly and have their conditions monitored, particularly women with rheumatic heart dis-ease. Doses over 150 IU daily are not usually recommended for rheumatic hearts. Before white flour became prevalent in 1910, stripping wheat of vitamins B-complex and E, heart and artery dis-eases were almost unknown.

Other uses for vitamin E include cold sores and to speed healing of all sorts, internally and externally, and removing and

preventing wrinkles and liver spots. It prevents muscular dystrophy in children when taken by pregnant women and is recommended in high doses for women with muscular dystrophy. Vitamin
E is positive for women who have migraines or visual problems,
especially eye muscle problems, difficult menstruations, PMS or
menopause difficulties, fibrocystic breast dis-ease, skin, hair or
muscular dis-eases, lack of sexual interest, internal or external
scars or keloids, bursitis and arthritis. Black women are especially
susceptible to keloids, high blood pressure and breast cancer, and
vitamin E (along with anti-racism) is a preventive.

Vitamin C is the anti-stress vitamin, highly important for
women in a patriarchal world. It's an antioxidant and antitoxin that
protects women's bodies from pollution and chemical toxicities. It is
listed as one of the four most deficient nutrients in women's diets
(with iron, calcium and vitamin B-2/riboflavin). Vitamin C prevents
and lessens colds (taking 1000 mg/l gm every hour at the first sign
of a cold or bladder infection may stop it) and is an anti-cancer
agent. Because it is water soluble, it is not possible to overdose with
vitamin C, though too much C can result in nausea, skin rash or
diarrhea. If this happens, decrease the dose to comfortable levels.
When using high doses of C, make sure to drink large amounts of
water to prevent kidney stones, or increase your magnesium intake.
I take vitamin C with a calcium-magnesium tablet for this, and also
take it at meals to prevent it from upsetting my stomach. Increase
vitamin B-complex and calcium when using megadoses of C for
longer than a few days. C reduces menstrual flows.

Women who are smokers and women living in polluted inner
city areas or near highways need increased amounts of vitamin C.
Aspirin triples the secretion rate of vitamin C, so alternate aspirin
with a C every couple hours if you use it. Taking vitamin C can alter
some laboratory tests—your practitioner should know you take it.
Avoid vitamin C if you are getting radiation or chemotherapy.
Vitamin C may prevent crib deaths (Sudden Infant Death Syn-
drome), and women who are nursing or on the pill need more of it.
Because vitamin C flushes from the body so quickly, a time-release
C is recommended.

Vitamin C has a thousand indications and benefits. It fights
bacterial and viral infections, colds, tonsilitis and ear infections,
and helps in gum dis-ease. It prevents and helps to treat hepatitis,
polio, diabetes, cataracts and eye infections, allergy and sinus
problems, ulcers, gallstones, even back problems. Vitamin C helps
blood circulation, prevents high blood cholesterol, athero and
arteriosclerosis, reduces blood clots/phlebitis, and strengthens the

blood vessel walls. It is useful in schizophrenia, joint dis-ease, anemia and bruising. Adele Davis relates:

> One physician gave a 45-year old woman with schizophrenia 1000 milligrams of vitamin C every hour, and at the end of 48 hours, by which time she had taken 45 grams, she was mentally well and remained so until she died some time later of cancer.[13]

Vitamin P or the C-complex bioflavinoids are recommended with vitamin C; they consist of rutin, hesperidin and citrin. The bioflavinoids are called the capillary permeability factor, and the capillaries are a filter that let nutrients through but stop viruses from entering the body. Symptoms for deficient Vitamin C and bioflavinoids include easy bruising, bleeding gums, excessive blood clotting, hot flashes, ulcers, asthma, edema and inner ear dizziness problems. Vitamin C works better with the C-complex, and there should be 100 mg of bioflavinoids for every 500 mg of vitamin C. A 1000 mg time-release C with bioflavinoids is your best bet daily.

The **B-complex vitamins** are a range of vitamin elements that all work together. No B vitamin should be taken alone, as each needs the rest of the complex to work at all. If deficient in any of these vitamins, take a full B-complex first and if more is needed, add the individual vitamin. Use with meals. These are all water soluble vitamins with no toxicity, but I have had severe nightmares after too much B-complex, probably from B-6. They disappear in a night or so after stopping the vitamin. A balanced B-complex is recommended for most women, especially vegetarians, plus a multiple vitamin that contains the full complex. Women with stress, depression, or mental/nervous disorders are strongly recommended for B-complex, or with migraines, PMS, epilepsy, candida albicans, asthma and allergies, or women who are on diuretics or antibiotics. Some women are energized by the B-complex tablets, but I use them at night for insomnia; different women react differently. Buy a B-complex that contains inositol, choline and folic acid, and hopefully PABA.

Vitamin B-1 (thiamine) aids digestion, mental attitude, the heart, muscles and nervous system. It helps with motion sickness and dental postoperative pain. Women who are pregnant, nursing or on the pill, women with multiple sclerosis, and women who smoke or have digestive issues need more B-1. Caffeine, alcohol, sugar, heat, estrogen, antibiotics and sulfa drugs destroy this vitamin in women's bodies. Shingles, brain damage, mental confusion, fatigue, heart dis-ease, central nervous issues, and numb hands or feet are other indications for thiamine.

Vitamin B-2 (riboflavin) is the most deficient vitamin in American diets. It is destroyed by light, particularly the light used to make vitamin D-enriched milk and by the refining of flour. B-2 is for stress, growth and helps prevent birth defects. It aids pregnancy, vision and eye fatigue, cataracts, anemia, digestive issues, oily skin, eczema, sores in mouth, lips or tongue, exhaustion, metabolism, and iron absorption. It prevents loss of hair, vaginal itching, depression, and is an anti-cancer agent. Most vegetarians are deficient in riboflavin, as are women on diabetic or anti-ulcer diets. Some cancer drugs are reduced in effectiveness by taking B-2.

Niacin or **vitamin B-3** is a major anti-stress and anti-migraine vitamin for women. A dose of 50 mg niacin every 10–15 minutes at the early start of a migraine can circumvent it, but it must be niacin and not niacinamide. Heating, flushing and reddening of the skin caused by increased circulation is sometimes experienced when taking niacin. The effect is strange, occurring only in women who are B-3 deficient, but it disappears in about twenty minutes. This flushing is what stops the migraine. Only one or two tablets are usually needed—take them every ten minutes or so until you get this flush.[14] Women without migraine issues can use niacinamide and avoid the flushing sensation.

Vitamin B-3 is essential for a healthy nervous, circulatory and digestive system. It reduces high blood pressure and bad breath, eases vertigo, headaches, constipation and diarrhea. It is used for schizophrenics and autistic children; hostility, personality changes and paranoia are B-3 deficiency symptoms. Backaches and insomnia are also indications for niacin.

Vitamin B-5 (pantothenic acid) is a major help for women who are hypoglycemic or suffer from adrenal fatigue. It is also a natural stimulant without side effects that I use regularly when travelling. Pantothenic acid is important for women with any sort of stress issues or stress dis-eases. I use 500 mg capsules twice a day with meals, increasing to as much as 2000–3000 mg a day if needed. Excess is released through the urine and there are no side effects, beyond too much energy. Avoid this one close to bedtime to prevent insomnia.

Velma Keith and Monteen Gordon in *The How To Herb Book* stress the need for pantothenic acid by reporting a Japanese study. Methyl bromide, a common tasteless insecticide used widely by food wholesalers, is reported to destroy B-5 in the items sprayed with it, changing it to an unknown compound.[15] If you are a vegetarian, as I am, pantothenic acid may be necessary for you. This is a major stress vitamin for the entire endocrine system.

Signs of B-5 deficiency include duodenal or stomach ulcers, headaches, hair loss, allergies or hay fever, respiratory or skin disorders, eczema, motor coordination impairment, anemia, AIDS, cataracts, thyroid problems, hypoglycemia, hypoadrenia, furrowed tongue, arthritis, postoperative shock and fatigue. Arthritis and allergies may be deficiency dis-eases of B-5. For allergies, take 1000 mg each of B-5 and C twice a day with meals. It is a natural antihistamine and immune system stimulant.

Barbara Seaman blew the whistle on **vitamin B-6** (pyridoxine) deficiencies in contraceptive pill users as the cause of phlebitis/blood clots and a number of women's deaths. B-6 is necessary for pill users and is also an aid to pregnant women for morning sickness, leg cramps and toxemia. It is also an aid for PMS anxiety and water retention. B-6 should not be used by women taking l-dopa for Parkinson's dis-ease, but arthritic women on cuprimine need increased amounts of it. This vitamin is positive for women who are hypoglycemics, epileptics, or have heart conditions, ulcers, kidney stones, anemia, arteriosclerosis, AIDS, rheumatism, diabetes (check blood sugar levels frequently, it may decrease insulin need), insomnia and for difficulties of menstruation or menopause. Nervousness and irritability, muscular or general weakness, and reduced immunity are other deficiency signs for B-6. Overuse can cause nightmares, but the vitamin is water soluble and nontoxic. Use no more than 50 mg a day if pregnant.

Vitamin B-9 is also called folic acid. It was restricted by the FDA for a time to tablets containing 0.1 mg with the government reasoning that folic acid use can mask vitamin B-12 anemia, but is now available in larger doses. Both B-9 and B-12 are important for long-term vegetarians. Folic acid deficiency is common among women, especially vegetarian or pregnant women. It is also important for preventing birth defects and hemorrhaging of the mother in delivery. It is helpful in menstrual difficulties, nursing, or any debilitated state. B-9 helps in tissue repair, regeneration, increases intelligence and prevents greying hair (with B-5). It is used to treat AIDS, atherosclerosis, dropsy, schizophrenia, catatonia and insomnia. Most vegetarians need it, also women who use alcohol, estrogen, dilantin, sulfa drugs or mega-vitamin C.

Vitamin B-12 (cyanocobalamine) may also be deficient in long-term vegetarians. Deficiency symptoms (experienced all at once) include reduced sensory perception, jerky limb motion, arm and leg weakness, and trouble walking and speaking. Not assimilated well by mouth, it is usually given in injections by doctors, but can be taken under the tongue in some forms. B-12 is also useful to women with difficult menstruation, nervousness, hormone use, memory loss, insomnia, depression, fatigue, anemia, some skin problems, bronchial asthma, schizophrenia, heart palpitations, abdominal difficulties, problems of pregnancy and lactation. I tried a B-12 and folic acid combination, knowing I need them, but it left me too constipated to continue using it. Try increasing fiber and liquids, or a carob milkshake twice a day to relieve this. B-12 in sublingual form is less constipating.

Vitamin B-13 (orotic acid) metabolizes B-9 and B-12, but is not readily available in the United States, except in better combination vitamins. It may aid in multiple sclerosis. More research is needed.

Vitamin B-15 (pangamic acid) is a Russian discovery that the FDA would like to take off the market. It prevents some glandular and nerve disorders, and is an antioxidant against pollutants. It may be a source of help for women in sobriety as it reduces alcohol cravings and protects against cirrhosis of the liver. It stimulates immunity and increases cell life, and is helpful in angina, asthma, high cholesterol and fatigue. Most forms are not available in this country. It is a water soluble vitamin with no toxicities.

Vitamin B-17 (laetrile) is another FDA banned vitamin under great controversy. Proponents value it as a cancer cure; detractors say it is toxic and worthless. It is made from the high cyanide-content kernels of apricot pits, apple seeds and other fruit seeds. Women who are interested in this treatment should seek the help of a nutritionist or nutritionally oriented, holistic physician. Suggested use is five to thirty apricot kernels through the day, not at once. More research is needed, but does not seem to be forthcoming from the FDA. Cancer is a multi-million dollar business for male medicine, and women its most frequent victims.

Biotin is another B-complex vitamin, sometimes called vitamin H. It is present in breast milk, and may be a reason why breast fed babies are healthier than bottle fed ones. Women who take estrogen, who are pregnant or nursing may be deficient, as well as women on antibiotics or sulfa drugs, or those who eat raw eggs (as in eggnogs) regularly. Seborrhea, eczema, dermatitis, dry peeling skin or cracked lips may be symptoms of biotin deficiency. Extreme fatigue and hair loss are biotin deficiency symptoms, as are heart dis-ease, muscle pains, depression, and insomnia. Biotin is necessary for metabolism of proteins, fats and carbohydrates in women's bodies. Most B-complexes and good multiple vitamins contain some amount of biotin.

Choline and **inositol** together make **lecithin**, and are B-complex vitamins. Choline is a fat emulsifier that helps to prevent arterio- and atherosclerosis, heart failure, gall bladder problems, and blood clots. It helps high blood pressure, glaucoma, leg cramps from constricted circulation, and improves memory. It is a help in multiple sclerosis and muscular dystrophy, Alzheimer's dis-ease, in diabetes, liver and kidney dis-ease, hepatitis and is an anti-cancer agent. It aids the thymus gland and spleen for immunity and red blood cell regulation.

Inositol is necessary for brain function and assimilation of vitamin C. Women after menopause need more of it, as well as heavy coffee drinkers or alcohol drinkers. It helps in athero- and arteriosclerosis to lower and control cholesterol levels, and in the assimilation and use of vitamin E for nerve damage. It is positive for women with cerebral palsy, multiple sclerosis and muscular dystrophy, helps vision and eye problems, gall bladder dis-eases, diabetes, skin and eczema issues, psoriasis, hair loss and some forms of mental retardation.

PABA (para-amino benzoic acid) is the last of the B-complex vitamins so far discovered, and is a part of the compound of folic acid (B-9). PABA aids in assimilation of protein and of pantothenic acid, and is destroyed in the body by sulfa drugs and antibiotics. PABA can make sulfa drugs ineffective and the FDA required a precription for its internal use for a while, but it is now available. Eczema is a PABA deficiency dis-ease, and digestive disorders, fatigue, depression and irritability may be PABA deficiency symptoms. PABA is useful for infertility in women, psoriasis, vitiligo, and intestinal health. It helps delay the effects of aging—wrinkles, liver spots, greying hair. A major commercial use for PABA has been as a sunscreen and protection from skin cancer. It greatly reduces the pain of burns. Commonest doses are 30–100 mg three times a day when used internally. PABA should be included in your multiple vitamin or B-complex tablet.

Vitamin F (essential fatty acids) is used with vitamin E as an antioxidant to clean up the free radicals formed by saturated fats. Free radicals are oxidants that damage cells. Vitamin F is a factor in reducing cholestrol and heart dis-ease, and also a protection against x-ray damage. The vitamin, composed of three items—linoleic acid, linolenic acid and arachadonic acid—influences the endocrine glands, especially the adrenals and thyroid. Skin dis-eases such as acne or eczema are vitamin F deficiencies, as are dry skin, dry dull hair, dandruff, diarrhea, gallstones, varicose veins and the loss of beneficial intestinal bacteria, as in colitis. Vitamin F aids respiration, nerves, reproduction, the skin and heart and regulates blood coagulation. In right amounts for the individual woman, it can cause weight loss, but an excess causes weight gain; there are no toxicities. Vitamin F's major uses are to reduce cholesterol and help the skin. Use with vitamin E and at meals for best results.

Vitamin K is usually available by prescription only, though natural forms of this fat soluble vitamin are nontoxic. Improper blood clotting, internal bleeding or excessive external bleeding are signs of vitamin K deficiency. The vitamin is sometimes prescribed before surgery and births to prevent hemorrhages, and for excessive menstrual flow. It is used in treatment of heart attacks. Other deficiency symptoms are colitis, excessive diarrhea, nosebleeds and celiac dis-ease. Alfalfa contains natural vitamin K (and most other vitamins and minerals), as does organic yogurt. X-rays, radiation, aspirin, air pollution, mineral oil, antibiotics and frozen or irradiated foods destroy it in the body. Without these, vitamin K deficiencies would be rare.

Vitamin U is important for healing ulcers, but little else is known about it, and the substance may not really be a vitamin. Again, more research is needed. Write your congressperson.

Unlike vitamins, minerals are inorganic; they cannot be made in women's bodies as most vitamins, but must be absorbed through food. Plants get them from the soil, and animals get them from plants. Though the amounts of most minerals in women's bodies is very small, the soil that provides them is increasingly depleted and is highly imbalanced by chemicals. Minerals make up actual structures in women's bodies, especially the bones and teeth, and deficiencies cause serious weaknesses. Some minerals make vitamin assimilation possible, as calcium with vitamin D and zinc with vitamin A. A few minerals are toxic in excess, while others require a balance (as calcium, phosphorus and magnesium, or potassium and sodium) to be effective.

Sixty to eighty percent of ingested calcium is lost, and ninety percent of iron, so mineral supplements have to be much higher than the body actually needs. Chelation of minerals makes them easier to assimilate, using natural rather than synthetic compounds, and minerals are also best used (as are vitamins) with meals. Where mineral deficiencies are extensive, use of hydrochloric acid tablets and digestive enzymes helps their assimilation. The minerals are discussed briefly here, with emphasis on those most important for women. Major deficiencies involve the bones and teeth, and lesser ones include depression, insomnia, fatigue, skin and hair problems, muscle cramps, menstrual and stress issues.

Calcium is probably the most familiar of minerals for women, and must be used with half the amount of magnesium and phosphorus to be effective. Phosphorus is unusually high in American women's diets due to phosphate fertilizers and additives, and women seldom need more. A good calcium-magnesium combination that also contains traces of zinc, A and D—General Nutrition's Calcium-Plus—is a wonderful tranquilizer that I use at times for insomnia. Calcium was my first vitamin—I began using it in high school on another girl's suggestion that it would prevent the leg cramps and charlie horses that were keeping me up at night. It worked within a few days, and for many years the spasms started again every time I went off of it. Use calcium-magnesium as an antacid, but not directly after meals, as antacids of any sort effect digestion.

Almost every woman requires extra calcium: elders, children, pregnant or nursing women, infants, women who are hypoglycemic, have menstrual cramps, backaches, muscle pains or cramps, allergies or insomnia. Calcium is positive in any form of stress and for headaches and migraines, pleurisy, bone or tooth dis-ease, arthritis, and heart dis-ease. It lowers cholesterol, decreases pain, and helps normal blood clotting. Use it especially after having dental work (1000-4000 mg of calcium with vitamin D) to help the pain and to replace the calcium balance lost from the work and stress. Calcium is helpful in menopause and after menopause for preventing osteoporosis and arthritis. It is recommended for women with multiple sclerosis and muscle dis-eases. Sources disagree on possible toxicities of calcium; most say it is nontoxic in any amount, while others recommend doses of under 2000 mg a day. Some sources believe that women need calcium-magnesium supplements every day for life.

Chromium is present in the body in trace amounts. Diabetes and arteriosclerosis may be its deficiency dis-eases. It balances glucose tolerance and can help prevent diabetes and hypoglycemia. It lowers high blood pressure and retards cholesterol formation in the arteries and liver. Suggested dosages are 25-250 mcg a day, the higher doses for women who have diabetes or are over sixty-five. If you are a diabetic, monitor blood sugar levels carefully when taking minerals and vitamins. Use vitamin C with chromium.

Cobalt is a part of vitamin B-12 (cyanocobalamine) and is a possible deficiency for long term vegetarians. Obtain it through B-complex or B-12 to help prevent anemia.

Copper is a trace mineral usually obtained from foods. It helps in the assimilation of iron and vitamin C, but supplements can upset the zinc balance in women's bodies. Some multiple vitamin/ mineral supplements contain it, otherwise get it from unprocessed foods. Deficiencies are rare and doses of more than 15 mg a day can cause side effects.

Fluoride is a mineral supplied by fluoridated water, a process under controversy. Fluoridation helps prevent tooth decay and cavities but does nothing for gum degeneration, and the chemicals are probably harmful to the liver. It may also be a factor in osteoporosis in elder women.[16] Fluoride is seldom found in supplements, and if your water is fluoridated, you are more likely getting too much than too little.

Iodine is contained in iodized salt and fluoridated water. If it's included in your multiple vitamin and mineral tablet and if your thyroid is stable, supplements are probably not needed. Goiter, slowness and obesity are symptoms of deficiency, and some pregnant women may need extra. Iodine deficiency in pregnancy can cause cretinism in the infant. If using supplements, make sure they are natural rather than synthetic, and try getting enough iodine from kelp. The FDA restricted iodine, claiming toxicity, but 2400 mg have been given daily for as long as five years, even to children, with no ill effects.[17]

Iron is one of the two major vitamin deficiencies of women, (along with calcium), and calcium, vitamin C, copper and cobalt are needed for iron assimilation in women's bodies. Daily doses are suggested at 20-60 mg a day for women, the higher amounts in menstruation or after childbirth, and for elders and growing girls. Tea, coffee, phosphates, food additives and preservatives deplete iron from women's bodies, as does heavy menstruation, bleeding or hemorrhaging.

Iron deficiency symptoms include anemia, weakness and fatigue, debility, dizziness, irritability, brittle nails, gas, nausea after meals, itching, constipation or diarrhea, hair loss, heart palpitations, poor attention span, and low resistance to dis-ease. Organic iron is nontoxic in adults, but may be toxic in children. Use only organic iron supplements, called hydrolized-protein chelate, and avoid inorganic compounds (ferrous sulfate) as they are less assimilable and cause constipation. Vitamin E and inorganic iron should be taken at least eight hours apart, but organic iron does not interfere with vitamin E. Women who should not take iron supplements are those with sickle-cell anemia, thalessemia or hemochromotosis. Use it with care in pregnancy. Most women who menstruate can benefit from an iron supplement.

Magnesium is used with calcium to help the assimilation of both and is a mineral needed by most women. It is generally nontoxic, and is a calmative and great help in stress. Nervousness is a sign of magnesium deficiency, as is premenstrual craving for chocolate. A calcium-magnesium tablet is positive for indigestion, more so than antacids that deplete these minerals. Avoid any antacid or calcium-magnesium right after meals. This is a good supplement to take before bed. Magnesium prevents kidney stones and gallstones (use it when megadosing C; it helps bone, teeth and tissue growth, helps the nerves and lifts depression, increases energy, lowers blood pressure and helps to prevent heart attacks). Mental confusion, fast pulse and irregular heartbeat are magnesium deficiency symptoms. Alcoholics are usually deficient in magnesium. More magnesium is needed in pregnancy or lactation, and for women on the pill or taking estrogen. A calcium-magnesium supplement can help PMS symptoms and menstrual cramps and pain. Use with vitamin C to lessen flows. If you live in a hard water area, you probably need less magnesium. Magnesium needs vitamins A, C, calcium and phosphorus to work.

Manganese is necessary for use of the B-vitamins, C and E. Deficiency symptoms include poor memory, poor muscle coordination and reflexes, bowed bones, dizziness, hearing problems, tinnitus (ear noises), and high blood sugar. Women need this vitamin for issues of muscular weakness, multiple sclerosis, myasthenia gravis, epilepsy, diabetes, digestion or food assimilation problems, fatigue, irritability, central nervous system dis-eases and degenerative dis-eases such as Alzheimer's. Women who are pregnant or nursing may need more manganese, as well as women who are heavy milk drinkers or meat eaters. Dosages of 2.5 to 5 mg a day are suggested of this trace mineral, but toxicities are rare.

Molybdenum helps iron utilization, but very little is known about this trace mineral. Supplements are not recommended until more is known, but it is one of several minerals suggested for AIDS.

Phosphorus is a major component of bones and teeth, and is essential in controlling nerve function. The mineral is used as a chemical fertilizer and food additive; most women are not deficient, but in fact may be getting enough to upset the phosphorus-calcium-magnesium balance. Teeth and gum problems, poor bone growth, arthritis, poor appetite control, and overweight or underweight issues may be phosphorus deficiencies. Phosphorus is necessary for utilization of vitamin D, calcium and niacin, and too much iron or calcium can make phosphorus ineffective. Too much phosphorus causes the body to over-release calcium, and is a factor in osteoporosis. More women are deficient in calcium than in phosphorus and the balance is important. Phosphorus toxicity is unknown, but if you wish to take phosphorus, use it with calcium and magnesium, or use bonemeal with vitamin D as the supplement.

Potassium and sodium, like calcium and phosphorus, work in balance, and modern foods provide too much sodium. Fasting, diuretics, diarrhea, hypoglycemia, or severe stress can cause a potassium deficiency. Women with edema, hypoglycemia, hypoadrenia, allergies or high blood pressure may benefit from potassium, and women who use diuretics may be losing too much. Coffee drinkers, cortisone or alcohol users, and choco-holics may be losing too much potassium. Symptoms include continual thirst, tiredness, insomnia, poor reflexes, weak hearts, muscle weakness, constipation, hypoglycemia and poor breathing. Try drinking orange juice daily before supplementing.

Selenium works with vitamin E as an antioxidant and has been called the anti-aging vitamin. It is an anti-cancer agent, and a DNA/RNA activator. It alleviates hot flashes in menopause. Selenium deficiency may be a factor in strokes, heart dis-ease, skin problems, early aging, infertility, and muscular dystrophy. Dose recommendations are 50–200 mcg, and very high overdoses may cause toxicities. More research needs to be done; it could be a very important supplement for women.

Sodium is so pervasive in American food that most of us are overdosed. It is the major culprit in high blood pressure and strokes. Few or no women need sodium (salt) supplements, except in rare cases of heat exhaustion.

Sulfur is needed for good skin and hair, and there are many external sulfur skin creams. The mineral works with B-complex for body metabolism. If you are getting enough protein, you are probably getting enough of this trace mineral. Supplements are not usually available.

Vanadium is another trace mineral rarely supplemented. It is useful in lowering cholestcrol and preventing heart attacks. More research needs to be done here. Vanadium in inorganic forms can be toxic to women's bodies.

Zinc regulates body processes, forms insulin, and controls muscle contraction; it regulates the body's acid/alkaline balance and the flow of enzymes in the cells, and is a factor in the synthesis of DNA. Losses occur in sweating, pregnancy and nursing. Down's Syndrome may be caused by zinc deficiencies in the mother. Elder women need more zinc, as do those after surgery or bleeding, girls at all stages of growth, and pregnant women. A signal of zinc deficiency is white spots on the fingernails. Extra zinc may require extra copper, as zinc uses it up. Zinc is nontoxic but doses over 150 mg per day are not recommended.

Zinc is positive for women with dry scaly skin or skin rashes, hair loss, skin sores, growth problems, too slow healing of wounds, acne or poor night vision. I use it for some of these things and for dandruff, which disappears while I use it. Zinc helps resist infections, increases immunity, reduces body odors, helps prevent diabetes, and reduces senility and inflammations. Use it for the hair, nails, eyes and skin, for poison ivy, infertility, schizophrenia, AIDS, Alzheimer's, hypoglycemia and for loss of sense of smell. Arteriosclerosis may be a zinc deficiency dis-ease, and Down's Syndrome. Use zinc in chelated natural form, with vitamin A. Women with irregular menstrual cycles may benefit from zinc, and women taking B-6 for menstrual issues may need more of it. Your daily multiple vitamin/mineral tablet should include zinc, and at least 15-25 mg a day is needed by most women.

As soils become more depleted and chemicalized, deficiencies and imbalances of trace and larger quantity (calcium, magnesium) minerals will continue to increase. While the emphasis in wholistic healing has been primarily on vitamins, minerals are receiving and will continue to receive more and more attention. That so many of these elements are indicated to prevent heart and artery dis-ease, degenerative dis-eases and high blood pressure/strokes shows how mineral deficiencies, soil depletions and chemical additives have created these dis-eases in modern women that were almost unknown less than seventy-five years ago.

I have used vitamins for more than twenty years and firmly believe in them. A good diet/good nutrition is essential, but is mostly not available to women today, and vitamins make up some of the losses. Healing results can take a longer time to show improvement, up to several months, but most results come sooner. Vitamins are a long-term way to help build women's well-being. For general health, use a well-balanced, good quality multiple vitamin and mineral supplement before adding other supplements. Taken with each meal on a good diet, the multiple may even be enough, but it won't be for many women. Use muscle testing or pendulum procedures to help you pick what you need, as every woman is different, and monitor changes over time. Retest every couple of months to see if the supplements and doses are still right for you or need revising.

Vitamins are one of the alternative therapies being used for **AIDS**, including megadoses of vitamins C, A, E, B-complex and zinc. At *least* 10,000 mg (10 gm) of vitamin C with bioflavinoids is used a day, up to 25,000 mg intravenously. The C is taken as a powder in liquids six times a day, sometimes in time-release, and usually in the non-acid calcium ascorbate form. If diarrhea occurs, reduce the dose. For vitamin A, the amount is 25,000–50,000 IU per day, usually as beta carotene/pro-vitamin A which is nontoxic. A maintenance dose of about 25,000 IU is suggested. Zinc amounts are about 100 mg a day, with 400–800 IU of vitamin E. A B-complex-100 is taken three times a day and a multiple vitamin/mineral supplement. Folic acid is supplemented to about 400 mcg, B-6 at 100–200 mg, extra B-12 to 500 mcg a day, extra biotin to 500 mcg, and 500–1000 mg of pantothenic acid/B-5. If stopping any of these large amounts, decrease them slowly. These vitamins and dosages are positive for any immuno-deficiency dis-ease. Minerals suggested include, besides zinc, iron 20 mg, copper 1–2 mg, manganese 10–20 mg, magnesium 300–500 mg, selenium 100–200 mcg, molybdenum 100 mcg, chromium 500 mcg, and germanium, all daily.[18]

For **arthritis**, Adele Davis suggests a high protein anti-stress diet, including lots of vitamins C, pantothenic acid and B-2.[19] Along with the multiple vitamin and mineral supplement, try 1000 mg of C and bioflavinoids three times a day with meals, B-complex-100, B-12 up to 2000 mcg daily, niacinamide up to 1000 mg/1 g, pantothenic acid/B-5 100 mg three times a day, and cod liver oil (A and D) one to two tablespoons or three capsules three times a day (use five days, skip two days).[20] Vitamin B-6 may be a preventive for rheumatism.

For **colds**, fevers and flu, at first symptoms start with 1000 mg of Vitamin C an hour, along with a calcium-magnesium tablet. Use a C that includes bioflavinoids, and when megadosing C drink lots of water. Decrease gradually. Another cold stopper is vitamin A, 25,000 IU hourly, 250,000 IU a day for up to three days. This works for some women when vitamin C doesn't, or try both. Either should end a cold within a day or lessen it greatly, but should be started as early as possible.[21] The vitamin C method also works for cystitis, the recurrent bladder and urinary infections some women are susceptible to. Use it along with a glass of *unsweetened* cranberry juice hourly.

For **menstrual** cramps and PMS, use vitamin C, 1000 mg time-release daily with bioflavinoids to decrease heavy flows. Use a calcium-magnesium supplement daily, not only during menses, to prevent PMS symptoms and menstrual cramps. These have worked very well for me, but it takes about three months to see real differences. Use a daily multiple vitamin and mineral supplement, 50 mg B-6, plus 400 IU vitamin E daily. Adele Davis suggests 5000 IU vitamin D daily and tablets at each meal of 250 mg calcium and 125 mg magnesium, taken for ten days before menses and during them,[22] to prevent cramps and PMS. The calcium-magnesium prevents some food cravings, particularly for chocolate, and lessens water retention. Also do affirmations, affirming your body and cycles. Women who celebrate, or own and honor their moon times have fewer or no PMS symptoms or other menstrual difficulties.

Vitamins for **menopause** include vitamin E and selenium, plus calcium-magnesium. Velma Keith and Monteen Gordon suggest 1000–1200 IU vitamin E, B-complex-50 with 50 mg B-6 and 250 mg B-5/pantothenic acid, and 50,000–75,000 IU vitamin A (try beta carotene or dry form).[23] Use 2000 mg calcium, 500 of magnesium, and 1000 IU of vitamin D daily.[24] The vitamin E will stop hot flashes and night sweats. Some E-complex preparations have selenium already in them.

For **migraines**, try 50 mg niacin at the very start every ten to fifteen minutes until the hot flush from the niacin dilates the blood vessels and ends it. Use niacin, not niacinamide for this, and a B-complex daily. If the headaches and migraines are premenstrual, calcium-magnesium and vitamin D may prevent them, also vitamins B-1 and B-12. Try B-6 and/or pantothenic acid daily. Most women who suffer from migraines are hypoglycemic and need pantothenic acid/B-5.[25] Eliminate chocolate, refined sugar and white flour products, eat several small high protein meals a day, and keep bowel movements regular. Work to reduce stress.

Pantothenic acid is the big one for **hypoglycemia**. Use 500 mg with meals twice a day, vitamin A and D capsules of 10,000 A and 400 IU D (I use double that), vitamin C 500 mg with each meal, vitamin E 100–200 IU three times daily, a B-complex-50 three a day (may be too much; if you develop nightmares and restlessness at night, decrease it), vitamin F, zinc, lecithin, chromium, and a multi-mineral/multi-vitamin tablet twice a day.[26] If you are subject to blackouts, try potassium.

For the **skin**, use vitamin E topically and internally to reduce scars and for burns. For rashes, psoriasis and eczema, vitamins E, A with D, zinc, vitamin F and lecithin are all positive. Use a multiple vitamin and mineral supplement and a B-complex-50. A, D and B-6 are used especially for acne, and if oil is a problem use the dry form A, D and E.

Suggested vitamins for **multiple sclerosis** are lecithin and vitamin F, with reduction in diet of saturated fats. Adele Davis says that early multiple sclerosis has been arrested with vitamins E, B-6 and B-complex in generous amounts. She suggests pantothenic acid/B-5 for stress, thiamine/B-1, riboflavin/B-2, lecithin and up to 1800 IU a day of E. Any muscular degenerative dis-ease calls for megadoses of E, including MS and muscular dystrophy.[27] In addition to these Velma Keith and Monteen Gordon suggest calcium-magnesium and all minerals, as well as mega amounts of vitamin A (use dry form). Remember to also use the multiple vitamin and mineral supplement.[28]

High blood pressure is increasingly a women's issue, and the multi-vitamin/mineral supplement is suggested, along with B-complex and megadoses of vitamins A, C with bioflavinoids, and E. Start with 100 IU a day of vitamin E, increasing it each month to a total of 400–600 IU daily. Do it slowly.[29] Kyolic (odorless garlic perles) is also very positive to reduce high blood pressure and cholesterol, as well as the Chinese herb dong quai (more on these next chapter). Other suggestions include lecithin, calcium-magnesium, and potassium (check with practitioner if you are on diuretics). Adele Davis suggests that a very small B-6 or choline deficiency can result in hypertension.[30]

For **insomnia**, B-complex and calcium-magnesium do wonders taken before bedtime. Use a multiple vitamin and mineral supplement with meals. Vitamin B-6 and niacinamide, 100 mg each before bed are a sedative, and also try 1000 mg alpha-tryptophan half an hour before bed.[31] Meditation for fifteen to twenty minutes nightly also works wonders.

For **vaginitis**, Adele Davis suggests 50,000 IU of vitamin A daily reduces vaginal inflammation and infections of the uterus, ovaries and fallopian tubes. With it use vitamins B-6, C, E and pantothenic acid/B-5. When megadosing A, try taking it for five days and stopping for two to prevent toxic buildups, or try the dry form. Vegetarians deficient in B-12 may develop irregular menstrual cycles and discharges with an odor that supplementing B-12 stops. Vaginal itching responds to B-2/riboflavin. Try a B-complex as vaginal issues can be deficiencies in any one of several B vitamins.[32] **Candida albicans**, recurrent or systemic yeast infections, often responds to acidophilus lactobacillus tablets that correct the imbalance of vaginal bacteria. Use these three times a day with meals. Kyolic may also be helpful and I recommend it.

To prevent **osteoporosis**, the thinning and demineralization of the bones that is primarily a women's dis-ease of later life, use calcium, magnesium and vitamin D. This should be started before menopause and continued throughout life, as lifelong mineral deficiencies are believed to be the cause. If your water is fluoridated, supplements are particularly necessary. Estrogen replacement therapy may slow the thinning of bone mass, but there are risks of cancer. Use a natural vitamin and mineral supplement, with 1000 mg daily of calcium and 500 mg of magnesium. Mega vitamins A, C, D, E and B-complex are also positive.[33] Barbara Seaman emphasizes calcium-magnesium, B vitamins, chromium and trace minerals.[34]

There are a number of excellent books written on vitamins and vitamin therapy; I suggest the ones referenced in this chapter. This chapter has been only a very brief introduction to vitamins and minerals, but should give women new to them a start. Vitamins were my own first healing method and I still use them extensively. I recommend them for their positive results. Use vitamins along with body-knowing and women's intuition to recognize your own needs and heal early symptoms.

NOTES

1. "Vital Vitamins", in *Light News*, (POB 770844, Houston, TX 72215), Vol. I, no. 3, March–April, 1988.

2. Dr. Harold Rosenberg, *The Book of Vitamin Therapy*, (New York, Berkeley Books, 1974), pp. 57–59. A disproportionate number of vitamin books were published between 1973 and about 1977.

3. *Ibid.*, p. 61.

4. *Ibid.*, p. 137.

5. Barbara Seaman and Gideon Seaman, MD, *Women and the Crisis in Sex Hormones*, (New York, Rawson Associates, 1977), pp. xi, 63, 155 and 287 ff.

6. Harold Rosenberg, *The Book of Vitamin Therapy*, pp. 137–141.

7. Prevention Magazine Staff, *The Complete Book of Vitamins*, (Emmaus, PA, Rodale Press, 1977), p. 9.

8. *Ibid.*, pp. 8–9.

9. Tony Webb, Tim Lang and Kathleen Tucker, *Food Irradiation, Who Wants It?*, (Rochester, VT, Thorsens Publishers, Inc, 1987), pp. 49–50, 54.

10. Prevention Magazine Staff, *The Complete Book of Vitamins*, pp. 9–10.

11. Velma J. Keith and Monteen Gordon, *The How To Herb Book*, (Pleasant Grove, UT, Mayfield Publishing Co, 1984), pp. 133–134. Recommended.

12. Suggested amounts are not RDAs, but dosages recommended by the referenced sources for this chapter.

13. Adele Davis, *Let's Get Well*, (New York, Signet Books, 1965), p. 124. Highly recommended.

14. Linda Clark, *Get Well Naturally*, (New York, Arco Publishing, 1982), p. 297.

15. Velma Keith and Monteen Gordon, *The How To Herb Book*, p. 104.

16. Barbara Seaman and Gideon Seaman, MD, *Women and the Crisis in Sex Hormones*, p. 317.

17. Adele Davis, *Let's Get Well*, p. 345.

18. Lawrence Badgley, MD, *Healing AIDS Naturally*, (San Bruno, CA, Human Energy Press, 1987), pp. 114–133. See Afterword in this book, also.

19. Adele Davis, *Let's Get Well*, pp. 108–109.

20. Earl Mindell, *The Vitamin Bible*, p. 232.

21. Linda Clark, *Get Well Naturally*, pp. 346–347.

22. Adele Davis, *Let's Get Well*, p. 247.

23. Velma Keith and Monteen Gordon, *The How To Herb Book*, p. 176.

24. Adele Davis, *Let's Get Well*, p. 250.

25. *Ibid.*, p. 277.

26. Earl Mindell, *The Vitamin Bible*, pp. 239–240.

27. Adele Davis, *Let's Get Well*, pp. 241–243.

28. Velma Keith and Monteen Gordon, *How To Herb Book*, p. 219.

29. *Ibid.*, p. 196.

30. Adele Davis, *Let's Get Well*, p. 213.

31. Earl Mindell, *The Vitamin Bible*, pp. 222–223.

32. Adele Davis, *Let's Get Well*, p. 249.

33. Velma Keith and Monteen Gordon, *How To Herb Book*, p. 221.

34. Barbara Seaman and Gideon Seaman, MD, *Women and the Crisis in Sex Hormones*, pp. 320–321.

Chapter Eight

———————◯———————

Using Herbs

If vitamins are one of the newest healing methods available, herbs are among the oldest healing methods known, going back to the matriarchies. They are time-tested and woman-tested, and are still a useful and powerful healing method today. Foremothers of the current abused drug industry, herbs were used and developed primarily by women in a mother to daughter line of oral tradition. They began with very early foraging cultures and tribes, where gathered plants were the mainstay of the food supply. Plants with medicinal properties were discovered, valued and used as the earliest healing. If the earliest healing relationships were midwife to birthing woman and mother to child, the earliest plant remedies were probably aids to childbirth and contraception, and remedies to help mothers and infants survive.

By the time of the matriarchies' decline, the herbal pharmacopia was established, based on information carried orally from generation to generation by mothers teaching their daughters. Earliest herbal remedies would have been simples, remedies using only one plant, as the effects of an herb are easiest to understand and follow when it is used alone. By the time of the Chinese *Nei Jing* the system was fully developed, and Chinese herbal healers used combinations of five to fifteen items, choosing from a traditional standard list of five hundred herbs. The tradition of Chinese herbals and recorded herb healing reaches back to 400 BCE. Herbs are the basis of the celebrated Chinese healing system, more so than acupuncture or any other method, and the modern herbal pharmacopia in China now contains almost 6000 entries.[1]

Herbs were also studied elsewhere and used for healing. Judy Chicago, in her Heritage Floor listings for The Dinner Party, names a number of early woman herbal healers. Earliest among them was

Queen Mentuhetop, from 2300 BCE Egypt, a ruler from the long line of Egyptian healer queens. Teachers of healers throughout the world, these women of Africa conducted the first medical schools of known recorded herstory. Zipporah, a Hebrew woman of 1500 BCE learned healing from Egyptian healer-queens at Heliopolis and brought the skills and learning home to her own culture.[2] Egyptian healing spread through Africa and the Mediterranean into Greece, Rome and across Europe, merging with the learning already known to healers of each culture.

In Greece, Agnodice (506 BCE) was the first western medical school-trained gynecologist, entering classes disguised as a man. By this time the patriarchy was established and women were not permitted formal education or the sanction of the male establishment. When it was discovered that Agnodice was a woman and a competitor, attempts were made to forbid her from practicing. The efforts to ban women from practicing medicine failed until the twelfth century, when the christian church forbade them. Aspasia of Athens was also a gynecologist and herbalist from the fourth century BCE.[3] Despite the practice of erasing the names of women from the records of patriarchal history, these women's names still remain.

Only a few women herbalists and healers are known from the ancient past. The dark ages of encroaching patriarchy and the church Inquisition were the reason for the loss in Europe. In Rome of the second and fourth centuries, before the church had reached full power, Aemilia and Metrodora were women known as healers, the latter for her written prescriptions for women's dis-eases, and dis-eases of the stomach and kidneys. Macrina, an early christian woman of Turkey in the fourth century, started a women's healing community and what was possibly the first hospital, based on herbal knowledge.[4] The early christian convents became seats of women's learning, havens for free scholarship, the only places where women could be educated and not forced to marry. Women herbal healers left records of their work for others to follow, establishing hospital-convent-learning centers throughout Byzantium and Europe. Women's freedom was curtailed in these convents by the twelfth century, but before women's learning was squelched there, Hildegard of Bingen (1098–1179) wrote her herbal and medical books that still remain. Her *Liber Simplicis Medicinae* was a manual of natural healing methods and herbs. It lists healing uses for 213 plants and 55 trees, plus mineral and animal-derived remedies. Laced solidly with charms and Goddess magick, this woman's book is considered the basis of today's western herbal learning and of the modern drug industry.⁵ From that time, women were forbidden the practice of medicine, the Inquisition began, and the line of women's healing tradition was destroyed.

Women were burned as witches from the 13th to the 17th centuries in Europe because they were successful healers, and competition to the new male-only medical schools and medical establishment. The witch-midwives had a sound knowledge of herbal healing and based much of their practice on it. Jacobe Felicie, born in 1292 in France, was a physician brought to trial for her success as a healer and forbidden to practice medicine. She escaped with her life. Geillis Duncan died in 1590 in Scotland for her skill as a healer, and there were many, many more who died.

The trials of healers held in America included Margaret Jones and Tituba, a Black slave woman. Tituba was eventually released from prison and sold, while Jones was the first woman to be executed for witchcraft in the United States.⁶ The open reason for Jones's trial was that she was competition to Massachusetts' male doctors because of her skill and herbal knowledge. Nine million women died in Europe and the United States (primarily in Europe), burned, hanged or drowned by the Inquisition, often for their medical knowledge. Their deaths broke but did not end women's oral chain of learning as witches and healers.

The witch-healers had a highly sophisticated knowledge of herbal healing and medicine. They used ergot to ease labor and shepherd's purse to prevent after-birth hemorrhaging. They used belladonna to stop uterine contractions in early pregnancy, and digitalis from the foxglove plant for heart dis-ease. Herbs were known to these women for contraception and abortion. They had herbal knowledge of painkillers, antispasmodics, tonics and cleansers, herbs for wound and infection healing, for digestion and fevers, and anti-inflammatory aids.⁷ Similar knowledge was known among women in cultures worldwide—in Africa, Native America, China and Asia, South America, the near and middle east. These women held the state-of-the-art medicine of their day, something male physicians did not. After the witch burnings had decimated the female and wiccan populations of the west, their learning was ridiculed, distorted and discredited by the church. Yet, like the Goddess religion and women's culture, the underground information passed from mother to daughter and survived.

Women today are still the practitioners and researchers of this skill that has been a women's healing skill since the matriarchies. Despite the takeover by men in the medical profession, and the takeover by big business of the drug industry that began with field-picked plants, women are still the main practitioners of herbal healing. This has remained true among rural women, but it has also grown into a movement-within-the-movement in women's spirituality. The Michigan Women's Music Festival has an herbal healing center, The Womb, organized by Billie Potts, and women come there to teach and be taught from all over the United States and the world. Other healers and healing centers have followed, and herbalism is no longer a legend but a skill of women's own. In the mainstream, the-back-to-land and New Age movements of the sixties and eighties have also revived herbal healing.

Herbs are as important today as they were in the past when they were the only remedies, with no other drugs. The witch/midwife/healer used her skill with herbs to save lives, to facilitate births and deaths, to regulate conception, and to ease women and children through every sort of dis-ease. Learning to use herbs is a method of survival for women in a misogynist patriarchal age. Their use keeps many women out of doctors' hands. Moreover, herbs are inexpensive and without side effects. They work more slowly and gently than chemical drugs and often heal dis-eases doctors can't. Herbs are powerful and empowering for women's healing.

Women of the past obtained their herbs from the fields, and their knowledge of them from their mothers and grandmothers. This chapter emphasizes use and assumes you have the herb available and safely identified. Today women in cities go to stores, botanicas and healthfood stores to buy herbs, and the price, though rising, is usually under a dollar an ounce for dried, identified, clean herb matter. Look for herbs that smell strong and are bright in color, as the fresher the herb the more potent. Always store herbs in a dark, cool, dry place, labeled carefully.

Herbs are used in several ways The most basic use is as a tea, also called a tissane. Pour boiling water over dried plant matter (leaf, flower or stem) and steep for five to thirty minutes. Herbs become bitter when steeped for longer than fifteen minutes, so ten minutes is fine. If you live in a fluoridated or chlorinated water area, distilled or bottled spring water is suggested for medicinal teas. It is best to cover the tea against light and escaping steam while steeping. Teas can be made in a cup or teapot; the water is boiled on the stove, then poured on the herbs away from flame. Weaker herb teas, using a teaspoon or two of herb to a cup of water, are used daily for chronic issues, for their vitamin/mineral content, or just because they taste good. For medicinal or acute dis-ease uses, I make my herbal teas quite strong (to near infusion strength), with at least two tablespoons of herb in the strainer basket that sits inside a mug-sized cup. Be careful not to pack the herbs too tightly. The basket is a small wicker strainer available from healthfood stores that holds the herbs. When the tea is steeped, lift the basket out, and drink the resulting strained herb tea. The herb amounts I give are for dried herbs; use three times as much if the plants are freshpicked. A wonderfully witchy thing to do is to return the used plant matter back to Goddess Earth with reverence and thanks.

When using a teapot, use a ceramic or enameled one, not exposed metal, as the chemicals of the herbs react unfavorably with the metal of the pot. Aluminum is particularly to be avoided in any form of cooking for its implications in Alzheimer's dis-ease. When making a pot of herbal tea for medicinal uses, use at least half a cup of dried herb matter for an eight cup teapot. Strain by pouring each cupful out through the herb basket, or strain the whole potful into another vessel. Herbs can remain in the pot for a while, though the brew can get bitter-tasting that way and they sour in a few hours. To keep a tea overnight, strain it and refrigerate; the tea can be reheated. The fresher made, the more potent for healing; never use a tea that has soured. Drink at comfortable temperatures.

Stronger teas are for acute healing issues when medicinal results are required. The stronger teas (see above) are near to infusion strength, and some sources would call them infusions, but a true infusion is slightly different. To make an herbal infusion, boil two cups (a pint) of water, and pour it over an ounce of herb matter. Let steep for six to eight hours, covered tightly. Billie Potts recommends using canning jars to make infusions, as they cover tightly and don't break with the heat.[8] Other jars or containers can be used, including stainless steel ones, but not plastic, aluminum or other metals. When these infusions are used at The Womb at the Michigan Women's Music Festival, the finished infusion is poured through a strainer to fill half a cup, with hot water poured over it to the top. For best results, keep the jars of steeping herbs in a dark place.

While softer plant parts—leaves, soft stems, flowers—are not boiled directly, woodier barks, stems, seeds, rhizomes and roots require boiling to bring out their properties. Such a preparation is called a decoction. The herb is placed in water in a pot on the stove, brought to a boil, and simmered for varying amounts of time. Some decoctions bring the water and herbs to a boil, then turn off the flame, letting the herbs steep for a few minutes or until cool. I used this method with a hair rinse combination (of yarrow, nettles and black walnut), pouring it into a pitcher with cool water to use after shampooing. Other herbs, such as valerian root, boil for a minute or two before taking off the flame.

A third type of plant decoction, described by Billie Potts,[9] is to simmer the herb in water until the amount of water has evaporated to half. A quart of water and two ounces of, say valerian root (a sedative herb), boils down to a pint (half a quart) of finished decoction. Another way of doing this is to boil an already made infusion down to half its water content, boiling the liquid only (not the infused herb matter). In using a decoction of this concentration, the dose is in tablespoonsful or half-cup amount, perhaps diluted in a cup of water for the taste, rather than two cups or more a day. Break up or powder the plant matter before putting it in the pot, to help release its medicinal properties.

Herbal tinctures (not water-based) are even more concentrated than decoctions. They require alcohol or cider vinegar. Alcohol works better, and since tinctures are taken by dropfuls in water, their actual alcohol content is minimal for alcohol-sensitive women. Tinctures take a long time to make, but they also last almost permanently if kept in dark glass bottles in a dark place. Women who use them keep a selection available at all times. To make an herbal tincture, place six to eight ounces of plant matter (some sources say four ounces) in a wide-mouth quart jar and fill to the top with 60 proof/30 percent or higher alcohol or apple cider vinegar. This makes a very large quantity of tincture. Some women make lesser amounts—use a ratio of one part herb to four parts liquid.[10] Let the mixture stand for three to six weeks (some sources say two weeks and recommend shaking the bottle night and morning), then separate the liquid from the herbs, squeezing out the herbs before returning them to the earth. Store the liquid, which is the tincture, in dark glass bottles with glass (not plastic) eyedroppers. (Plastic, like metals, reacts unfavorably with the herbs.) Use tinctures by the dropful; they are very concentrated. A commercial tincture I used for a while had directions to use six drops twice a day in water, others say five to fifteen drops. They are very powerful.

Herbs taken orally are also used in capsules, though they may not be as fully assimilated by the body that way as in liquid form. However, some herbs taste too bad to drink, like the cayenne pepper and goldenseal I use to head off colds. I put these powdered herbs into size 00 gelatin capsules, found at food co-ops and healthfood stores. To fill the capsules, mix the herbs in a flat bowl, then hold one end of the capsule in each hand and bring the ends together through the herb mix. Dust them off on a paper towel before using (cayenne burns the mouth). Commercial encapsulators are also available. I generally make up a bunch at a time, as the process is messy, and store them in a dark container. Herbs can be made into pills by rolling the plant powder into soft bread or cream cheese.[11] Herb tablets and capsules are often available in healthfood stores, but except for roots, I wonder about their freshness. Herbs meant to be sucked, as slippery elm for sore throats, are sold in lozenges. Most herbs are more effective taken in infusions, decoctions or tinctures than they are in capsules or pill form. Capsules or pills are useful when you need to take a lot of herbs. Drink a lot of water with capsules or pills to prevent overloading your kidneys.

For external use, herbs are made into poultices or compresses (also called fomentations), and into salves and oils. A compress is a cloth wet with a hot herbal infusion used on the skin. A poultice is a cloth with the moistened dried herb (the tea dregs) wrapped in it and placed on the skin. With fresh herbs, place the crushed herb leaf directly on the skin. Insect bites and poison ivy rashes respond wonderfully to poultices of comfrey leaf, plantain or jewelweed, and bee stings to a slice of raw cucumber, potato, squash or zucchini.[12] Naturopaths rely on hot poultices of onions, mustard, bran or clay to detoxify the body in various ills and congestions. They are wonderfully soothing.

Salves are another external use for herbs made by adding herb material to a beeswax base. Herb oils are also useful; herbs are added to an olive oil base for herb oils. An infused oil (as compared to an essential oil that requires distillation), is made by placing half to two pounds of herb in a quart jar, and filling the jar with olive oil, covering the plant matter completely. Close tightly and store in a dark place for three to six weeks. (Other sources say two to three weeks, shaking the bottle daily or twice daily.) Pour off the oil, removing the plant matter, and store the herbal oil in dark glass bottles. Return the plant matter to Goddess Earth. These make wonderful liniments and massage oils, and the same process is used to make herbal scents.

For salves, take three or four ounces of the herb oil, and heat it over low heat. Grate 1/8 to 1/4 ounce of beeswax into it, warming until the wax has fully melted. Pour onto a cool plate and, when hardened solid, scrape into small widemouthed jars kept from the light. This makes wonderful hand and skin cream. Try it with calendula or comfrey. Be careful not to overheat or burn the oil. To make a salve without first making the herbal oil, place the herbs covered with olive oil in a lidded oven casserole dish and bake at 200–250° F for two hours. Strain out the oil and bring it to the top of the stove, add the beeswax and proceed as above.[13] Salves can also be made with vaseline,[14] but vaseline is a petroleum product.

The beeswax and olive oil salve is totally natural and safe.

Herbal baths are made by adding a pint of infusion or decoction to a bathtub full of water and soaking in it. Strain it so the herbs don't clog the drain, or put the dried herbs in a loose-woven cloth pouch, hanging them over the faucet so the water runs through. Try an herbal bath for insomnia, using valerian, lime blossom or hops.[15] Herbal infusions can also be used as douches and are effective for vaginal infections. Goldenseal and myrrh, boiled as a decoction and cooled to body temperature is a good douche for stubborn vaginitis and yeast. Except where noted, the recipes come from Billie Potts' *Witches Heal*, a highly valuable herbal for women.

Traditionally, herbs are categorized by their actions, but the standard list of actions is not always clear to modern women. An herb can have more than one action and usually does. Women choose the herb that best fits their healing issue(s). While the trend today is to mix together a number of herbs in an infusion or decoction, it is simpler and probably more effective to use one or two that most closely fit your needs. Fourteen different herbs may be useful for treating urinary infections, but it's expensive and inconvenient to find and buy so many. Instead, pick one, two or three most suitable for the symptoms. There are a number of excellent books that are herb materia medicas, listing each herb and what it does; use these as a guide. Uva ursi is my own and many other women's choice for cystitis, if you don't use the cranberry juice and vitamin C mentioned in the last chapter. Also try yarrow or buchu. Here is a list of herb actions.[16]

Alterative: Herbs to change physical condition, blood cleansers. Burdock, echinacea, nettles, red clover.

Analgesic or anodyne: Herbs to relieve pain. Plantain, valerian, white willow, witch hazel.

Antibilious: Reduces bile (gall bladder, liver). Dandelion, goldenseal, mugwort, vervain.

Anticatarrhal: Dries the mucous membranes of sinuses, mouth, vagina. Echinacea, garlic, goldenseal, hyssop, sage, yarrow.

Anti-emetic: Herbs that reduce nausea and vomiting. Dill, fennel, meadowsweet, peppermint.

Anti-inflammatory: Reduces inflammations. Chamomile, marigold, St. John's wort, white willow, witch hazel.

Antilithic: Relieves urinary stones. Buchu, gravelroot, uva ursi.

Antimicrobial: Natural antibiotics. Echinacea, garlic, myrrh, peppermint, plantain, rosemary.

Antispasmodic: For cramping and muscle spasms. Black cohosh, chamomile, cramp bark, scullcap, thyme, valerian.

Aromatics and carminatives: Herbs that smell good and stimulate digestion. Dill, fennel, ginger, peppermint.

Astringent: Herbs that tighten skin and mucous membranes, reduce discharges. Bayberry, oak bark, plantain, raspberry, rosemary, slippery elm, yarrow.

Bitter: Bitter tasting herbs that stimulate digestion via taste. Boneset, chamomile, goldenseal, hops, white horehound.

Cholagogue: Stimulates bile. Barberry, dandelion.

Demulcent: Soothes internal irritations. Comfrey, slippery elm.

Diaphoretic: Promotes perspiration for colds and fevers. Cayenne, elder, garlic, ginger, peppermint, yarrow.

Diuretic: Increases urine, for urinary infections. Buchu, corn silk, dandelion, gravel root, parsley, uva ursi, yarrow.

Emmenagogue: Herbs to bring on and regulate menses. Black or blue cohosh, cramp bark, motherwort, parsley, pennyroyal, peppermint, raspberry, St. John's wort, valerian, yarrow.

Emollient: For external soothing. Chickweed, comfrey, marshmallow, plantain, rose petals, slippery elm.

Expectorant: Removes mucous from lungs and sinuses. Coltsfoot, comfrey, hyssop, mullein, white horehound.

Febrifuge: Herbs to lower fevers. Boneset, Cayenne, feverfew, hyssop.

Galactogogue: Increases breast milk. Aniseed, fennel, raspberry.

Hepatic: Herbs for the liver. Barberry, dandelion, yarrow.

Hypnotic: For insomnia. Hops, scullcap, valerian.

Laxative or Cathartic: Stimulates colon cleansing. Aloe, burdock, cascara sagrada, dandelion, senna, yellow dock.

Oxytocic: Herbs that stimulate uterine contractions in childbirth. Blue cohosh, goldenseal, squaw vine.

Pectoral: Respiratory healing herbs. Coltsfoot, comfrey, garlic, goldenseal, hyssop, mullein, white horehound.

Sedative: Relaxants. Black cohosh, blue cohosh, hops, red clover, scullcap, valerian.

Stimulant: Energizing. Bayberry, cayenne, gotu kola.

Vulnerary: Herbs for external wound healing. Aloe, chickweed, comfrey, jewelweed, plantain, slippery elm, St. John's wort.

There are herbs and herb combinations for most or all of women's healing needs. While it is not possible in a chapter to list many of the thousands of healing herbs, a few are described here that are used often by women. Again, the description has to be brief and incomplete. For further information on healing herbs read Billie Potts' *Witches Heal*, Velma Keith and Monteen Gordon's *How to Herb Book*, or David Hoffman's *Holistic Herbal*. The herbs that follow are used internally as infusions or decoctions, unless otherwise noted. They can also be made into tinctures.

Alfalfa is a major nutritional herb, as it contains vitamins A and K in high amounts, and virtually every vitamin and mineral. It also helps women to assimilate plant matter for healing. I have used alfalfa with burdock and white willow to ease arthritis. Use it for allergies, rheumatism, digestion, morning sickness and teeth. Alfalfa has a lovely taste.

Aloe Vera soothes and heals on contact for all external wounds, burns, abrasions, rashes and cuts. It's great for poison ivy. Use it by itself or with vitamin E on burns. Internally, this herb is a laxative and cleanser, and brings on menses. Avoid in pregnancy, as it may start contractions, and avoid when nursing. Make sure you get pure aloe vera, without additives, for internal use, and use only small amounts. (Capsules are recommended.) Keeping one of these plants in the house is many women's first step to herbal healing.

Black Cohosh is a natural estrogen, without the carcinogenic effects of synthetic drugs. Use it for menopause (with blue cohosh) and menstrual cramps, and to bring on menses (with ginger). It reduces uterine spasms, helps in childbirth pain and afterpain, high blood pressure and nervous disorders. It balances women's hormones.

Blue Cohosh is used to prevent miscarriage and false labor, and to start real labor when the time is right. It helps to dilate the cervix in childbirth. Use it for menstrual cramps, to bring on menses, for uterine problems, vaginal infections, cystitis, and also for rheumatism, allergic reactions to bee stings, epilepsy and colic.

Boneset is a highly bitter herb, considered the best possible for stopping flus and fevers; use it with cherry bark for sore throats with flu. An internal cleanser, it helps congested sinuses, rheumatism, broken bones, and uterine and liver issues. Try it as a tincture; it tastes bad.

Burdock clears toxins from the body. It is useful for any skin, allergy or arthritis issues, as well as kidney and bladder infections. It detoxifies the lymphatic system and has been used in anorexia nervosa. Use externally and internally for burns, eczema, acne, psoriasis, poison ivy or poison oak. Use it also as a laxative.

Chamomile, many women's first herb, is the gentlest and probably best known of herbs. Use it for infants' or adults' colic,

Single Herbs

Alfalfa Nourishes entire system. Good for pituitary gland. Alkalizes the body rapidly. Helps detoxify the liver. Helps rebuild decayed teeth. Relieves arthritic, rheumatic pain.

Aloe Vera Aloe Vera is a potent medicine and healer. An excellent colon cleanser. Healing and soothing to stomach, liver, kidneys, spleen, bladder. Excellent remedy for piles and hemorrhoids. Works with immune system to keep you healthy, strong and vibrant.

Bayberry Clears congestion from nose, sinuses. Tea is excellent as gargle for sore throats. Valuable for all kinds of hemorrhages.

Bee Pollen A miracle food from nature rich in vitamins, minerals and amino acids. Reduces or eliminates the craving for protein.

Black Cohosh Natural estrogen; helps relieve menopause systems. Good for high blood pressure (equalizes circulation). Helps relieve pain in childbirth.

Black Walnut Hulls Expels internal parasites, tape worms. Rich in manganese for nerves, brain and cartilage. Helps relieve many kinds of skin problems.

Burdock Cleanses and eliminates impurities from blood. Diuretic. Soothing to the kidneys.

Cayenne (Capsicum) Used as catalyst in herbal formulas. Equalizes circulation, stimulates heart, helps heal ulcers of stomach and colon. Combined with Lobelia, excellent for nerves.

Cascara Sagrada Very good remedy for gallstones, increases secretion of bile, and one of the best remedies for chronic constipation.

Catnip Excellent for small children with colic. Very good as a sleeping aid; soothing to nerves. Useful in allaying pain caused by spasms.

Chaparral Blood purifier. Helps acne, arthritis, chronic backache, tumors, warts, skin blotches.

Chickweed Used extensively to help lose weight. One of the best remedies for tumors, piles and swollen testes. Excellent bronchial cleanser. Heals and soothes.

Comfrey Root Good blood cleanser. Helps heal ulcers, kidney problems. Best remedy for blood in urine. Remedy for coughs, catarrh.

Damiana A great sexual rejuvenator. Gives new energy.

Dandelion Excellent for anemia because it is high in iron, calcium, vitamins and minerals. Diuretic. Useful in kidney, bladder problems.

Devils Claw Very effective for arthritis symptoms as well as liver and kidney problems.

Dong Quai Ancient Chinese herb referred to as female equivalent to Ginseng. Nourishs female glands, regulates monthly periods, rebuilds the blood, helps conditions in the mother after birth of a baby. Taken by men and women for eczema, hypertension and kidney disorders.

Eyebright Main herb for protecting and maintaining health of the eye. Acts as internal medicine for constitutional tendency to eye weakness. Removes cysts caused by chronic conjunctivitis.

Fennel Helps suppress the appetite. Aids in digestion when uric acid is problem. Good for gas, acid stomach, gout and colic in infants.

Fo-Ti Excellent for mental depression. Has been used to help the memory.

Garlic Stimulates activity of digestive organs. Emulsifies cholesterol; loosens it from arterial walls. Useful for asthma, whooping cough, intestinal infections. Reduces high blood pressure.

Ginger Excellent motion sickness aid. No sedative effects on central nervous system, unlike drugs. Helps absorb toxins, restore gastric activities to normal. Helps control diarrhea and vomiting that often accompanies gastrointestinal flu.

Ginseng, Korean Promotes mental and physical vigor, metabolism, appetite and digestion. Mildly stimulates the central nervous system.

Ginseng, Siberian Physical restorative. Regenerates, rebuilds sexual centers. Anciently known as a male hormone, and used for longevity.

Golden Seal Herb Contains many of the same properties as the root but in milder form. Relieves nausea. Infusion makes a good vaginal douche. Used as an antiseptic mouthwash.

Golden Seal Root A powerful agent used in treating ulcers, diphtheria, tonsillitis and spinal meningitis. One of the best substitutes for quinine. It acts as an insulin.

Gotu Kola Contains remarkable rejuvenating properties. Known as "The Secret of Perpetual Youth." Strengthens heart, memory and brain.

Horsetail (Shavegrass) Contains a great deal of silica, which helps keep the elasticity in the skin. Also a diuretic. Helps with kidney stones.

Kelp, Norwegian Excellent for thyroid gland, goiters. Has a remedial, normalizing action on sensory nerves. Good for nails, hair, radiation.

Licorice Root Natural cortisone. For hypoglycemia, adrenal glands, stress, coughs, chest complaints, gastric ulcers, throat conditions.

Lobelia Powerful relaxant. Reduces palpitation of the heart and strengthens muscle action. Good for fevers, pneumonia, meningitis, pleurisy, hepatitis and peritonitis. Emetic in large amounts.

Parsley Rich in vitamin B and potassium. Excellent diuretic. One of the best herbs for gall bladder problems. Expels gallstones.

Pau D'Arco Greatest treasure the Incas left us. Possesses antibiotic, tumor inhibiting, virus killing, antifungal, anti-malarial properties. Effective for anemia, asthma, psoriasis, colitis. Aids resistance to various infections by building the immune system.

Psyllium Excellent colon cleanser, cleans out compacted pockets. Creates bulk. Relieves auto-intoxication.

Red Clover Blood purifier. Contains silica, other earthy salts. Relaxing to nerves, entire system.

Red Raspberry Tea is excellent for morning sickness. Helps prevent miscarriage; strengthens uterine walls prior to giving birth.

Saffron Natural hydrochloric acid (utilizes sugar of fruits and oils), thus helping arthritics get rid of uric acid which holds the calcium deposited in joints. Also reduces lactic acid build up.

Sarsaparilla Eliminates poisons from blood and helps cleanse system of infections. Useful for rheumatism, gout, skin eruptions, ringworm, scrofula, internal inflammation, colds, catarrh.

Scullcap More effective than quinine, and not harmful. Good for neuralgia, aches and pains, nervous tension. Helps reduce high blood pressure, helps heart conditions and disorders of the central nervous systems such as palsy, hydrophobia and epilepsy.

Slippery Elm Very valuable for inflammation of the lungs, bowels, stomach, kidneys and bladder. Will soothe ulcerated or cancerous stomach when nothing else will.

Uva Ursi Useful in diabetes, kidney troubles. Excellent remedy for piles, hemorrhoids, spleen, liver, pancreas, gonorrhea. Also good where there are mucus discharges from the bladder with pus and blood.

Valerian Root Nerve tonic. Used for epileptic fits, nervous tension or irritations. Promotes sleep. Excellent for children's measles, scarlet fever.

White Oak Bark Good for varicose veins. Used in douches and enemas for internal tumors, swellings. One of the best remedies for piles, hemorrhoids, hemorrhages or any trouble of the rectum. Normalizes the liver, kidneys and spleen.

White Willow Bark Nature's aspirin. Excellent as a pain-relieving, fever-lowering, anti-inflammatory agent without any side effects. Helps relieve symptoms of headache, fever, arthritis, rheumatism, bursitis, dandruff, eye problems (eyewash), influenza, chills, eczema, and nosebleed. Most effective in concentrated extract form.

Yellow Dock Mineral rich plant, high in iron. Excellent blood purifier. Tones entire system.

Yucca New hope for arthritics. Has been used with surprising success for arthritis and rheumatism symptoms.

insomnia, stress or anxiety. It helps in regulating menstruation and brings on menses; use it with raspberry leaf for cramps. Chamomile reduces inflammations and spasms. It is also used as a sore throat gargle and eyewash. It helps circulation, headaches, and drug withdrawals. A few women are allergic to it.

Coltsfoot is a respiratory herb for coughs, bronchitis, emphysema, chest congestions and asthma. Use it rolled in a cigarette smoked to draw in the fumes, drink it in infusions, and/or apply it as an external poultice. It is good externally for boils and skin ulcers, and internally for cystitis. It is very high in zinc.

Comfrey is almost an all-healer, high in calcium, vitamins C, A, B-12 and chlorophyll besides. Use it for coughs and infections including streptococcus, for colitis, internal ulcers, hemorrhages, varicose veins, and externally for bruises and wounds. It is useful in cystitis, yeast and vaginal infections, heavy menstrual flows and herpes. Lung and respiratory issues respond to comfrey, also pneumonia, arthritis, urinary or kidney stones, sore throats, rheumatic joints and broken bones. Use externally for insect bites, athlete's foot and skin rashes.

Damiana is an herb some sources list for men, but others list as positive for almost all 'female problems.' Use it as a hormone balancer particularly in menopause, for hot flashes, cystitis, and for women's infertility. The herb is an antidepressant, laxative and tonic. It is also used for Parkinson's dis-ease.

Dandelion contains potassium, calcium, cell salts, vitamins A, B-complex, C and E. It is traditionally used for gallbladder, spleen, urinary, kidney and women's reproductive issues. Use it as an internal cleanser and laxative, and for acne, eczema, cystitis, diabetes, arthritis, asthma, low blood pressure, Alzheimer's and hypoglycemia. Pick this herb outside in a clean place.

Dong Quai (tang kwei) is a female toner and hormone balancer. Use it for menstrual regulation, cramps, PMS, ovarian cysts, menopause, hot flashes, breast abscesses, and in pregnancy. This Chinese herb is a tranquilizer and balances both high and low blood pressure and blood sugar levels. It helps migraines, stroke recovery and internal injuries. It is also slightly laxative. Dong Quai is becoming quite popular in the women's healing community.

Echinacea is a natural antibiotic for bacterial and viral diseases. I have used it to help tonsilitis and lymphatic issues, as well as strep throats and swollen glands. Billie Potts recommends it for blood poisoning, pneumonia and herpes. She cautions that treatment has to be continued long enough, and that the herb should be saved for serious issues and not overused. Use it also for pelvic inflammations and mastitis, cancer, AIDS, wounds and fevers, and with yarrow in cystitis.

Ephedra (Ma Huang) is another Chinese herb for women's healing, useful for asthma, bronchitis, hayfever, allergic reactions and whooping cough. It increases blood circulation and is useful for low blood pressure.

Eyebright is known primarily as an eyewash for dis-eases of the eye and vision, including infections and conjunctivitis. It is also positive for hay fever and sinus issues, allergies, for digestion and gallbladder, and to calm the nerves. This is a potent decongestant used for many of the same things as the overused and expensive goldenseal.

Feverfew is becoming known for preventing migraines; four little flowers or a teaspoon of the dried herb as a preventive tea is taken daily. It is a vasodilator, relaxant and anti-inflammatory used for acute arthritis, painful menstruation and PMS. It increases menstrual flows. It helps ear noises (tinnitus) and dizziness. Avoid in pregnancy as it may cause uterine contractions. I have used feverfew for migraines with success and recommend it to others.

Garlic (Kyolic, odorless garlic perles) is a natural antibiotic for bacterial, viral and fungus infections and is an anti-cancer agent. It reduces high blood pressure and cholesterol levels. Use garlic for recurrent colds and flu, lowered immunity, AIDS, asthma, respiratory issues, hypoglycemia, colitis, arthritis, chronic bronchitis, tonsilitis and coughs. It combines well with echinacea and is very powerful and positive, very useful in reducing high blood pressure and artery dis-ease in women. It contains vitamins A, B-complex, C and most minerals.

Goldenseal is another natural antibiotic, probably overused by women and highly expensive. Use it with myrrh or cayenne in capsules to head off a cold, two capsules every three hours. Taken early enough, it will prevent a cold if used for the cold-type (chilled), rather than hot-type (fevered) colds. As a douche, use goldenseal and myrrh for yeast or other vaginal infections. Use it internally and externally for skin cancer, septic ulcers, colitis, heavy menstrual flows and hemorrhages. It is an aid to uterine contractions in labor but is also an abortifacient not to be used in a wanted pregnancy before term. Goldenseal is an all-healer, but hypoglycemics may have trouble using it as it lowers blood sugar.

Hops is a sedative and painkiller, for insomnia, shock, headaches and migraine pain, for PMS tension, and for anxiety and nervous system dis-eases. I used it regularly with scullcap and catnip for recurrent migraines before I knew about feverfew. It is useful for colitis and ulcers, cramps, indigestion, and improves the liver and gallbladder. Alcohol tinctures (not water infusions) are positive for strep infections, skin inflammations and abscesses. Avoid using hops for depression—it may aggravate it.

Hyssop is an antispasmodic useful for sore throats, lung congestions and fevers. I use it with echinacea for these issues. It is also an antibiotic. It brings up mucous in colds, coughs and bronchitis, and is positive for asthma and petit mal epilepsy. It normalizes blood pressure, and helps circulation. Use it with white horehound and coltsfoot for coughs and bronchitis, with peppermint, boneset and elder flower for colds. Hyssop will stop or limit a sore throat if used early enough, the key to most treatments.

Licorice Root is a natural estrogen, useful for women's menstrual cycles and menopause without side effects. It is an adrenal stimulant and natural cortisone for Addison's dis-ease, arthritis, diabetes, Epstein-Barr Syndrome, and hepatitis. Use it especially for hypoglycemia. Licorice is used in treating stomach ulcers, colic and gastritis, as well as bronchial dis-eases, emphysema and coughs. It is a mild laxative, and is used to help hoarseness, injured voices and voice muscles. It strengthens the heart and circulatory system, but can raise blood pressure.

Motherwort is a women's healing herb for bringing on menses, menopause issues and easing false labor. It relaxes the muscles in childbirth, and is used primarily a few days after delivery to empty the uterus and prevent infections. It regulates menstrual cycles and prevents cramping. The herb is also known as a heart remedy for rapid heartbeat and anxiety-caused dis-comfort. Use it for insomnia, rheumatism, sciatica and to regulate blood pressure. Avoid during pregnancy and immediately after delivery.

Nettles is a diuretic and tonic, a blood cleanser and skin and hair herb. Use it with burdock for eczema and psoriasis, and with burdock, yarrow and black walnut (or rosemary) for scalp and hair dis-eases. Nettles helps PMS water retention and adds iron and calcium; it is a lymphatic cleanser and releases urinary/kidney stones. Use it to stop internal bleeding including postpartum hemorrhaging and bleeding from the lungs, stomach or urinary tract. It helps headaches and is positive for the heart. Nettles is anti-inflammatory and helps to lower blood sugar levels. Use it moderately to prevent over-urination and kidney strain.

Parsley is used for urinary tract infections and kidney issues. It is a diuretic containing iron, potassium, vitamins A, B and C, and is a cancer preventive and immune system stimulant. Parsley is recommended as a menstrual regulator, to bring on menses, and as a hormone balancer for menopause; it contains natural estrogen. It is good for the adrenals and pituitary, for the nervous system, digestion, assimilation and elimination. For swollen glands, drink one or two cups of parsley tea at the first sign and a cup every two hours as needed. Avoid parsley in a wanted pregnancy, as it can cause uterine contractions and miscarriage.

Pau D'Arco (Taheebo, Lapacho) is a new herb for women, drawing considerable attention as an all-healer. It's an anti-cancer agent that stimulates the immune system, with implications for AIDS, lupus, multiple sclerosis, colds and flu. It has shown positive for candida albicans (recurrent or systemic yeast infections), herpes, cystitis, leukemia, psoriasis, Parkinson's dis-ease, rheumatism, ulcers and asthma. It is anti-viral, anti-fungal and anti-malarial, helpful in skin dis-eases, gastritis, colitis, for inflammations, tumors, wounds and pain.[17]

Peppermint is wonderful for gas, colic, nausea and indigestion. Chewed fresh, placed as an essential oil on the temples, or sipped as a tea it can stop headaches and early migraines. It is both a stimulant and relaxant (nervine) and, taken with elder flowers, boneset or yarrow can stop the flu. Peppermint is used for menstrual cramps, PMS tension, morning and travel sickness, to relieve fevers, colitis, dysentery and diarrhea. It calms the nerves, helps dizziness and fainting, aids colds, and slows heart palpitations.

Raspberry Leaf is the most basic herb for women's menstrual and pregnancy issues. Use it to regulate cycles, with chamomile for PMS and menstrual cramps, and to decrease heavy flows. It brings on menses and aids urinary infections. In pregnancy, raspberry tea is used throughout to ease morning sickness, aid labor, prevent hemorrhaging and afterbirth pain. It helps to prevent miscarriage and increases breast milk. Raspberry helps digestion, lowers fevers, stops diarrhea, mouth and stomach ulcers and is useful for vaginal discharges. It is good tasting, and useful for colds, measles and coughs.

Red Clover is a mild herb known for skin uses, and also used with violet is an anti-cancer and anti-tumor agent. Use it with violet to reduce or eliminate ovarian or uterine cysts, drinking half a pint in the morning and half again in the evening over a six-month period. Use one ounce of herb mix to a pint of water. In skin health, red clover is a wash for sores. It is used in children's or women's acne, eczema or psoriasis. For women recovering from debilitating dis-eases like mononucleosis or anemia, clover is a tonic and blood purifier. It's useful for coughs, whooping cough and bronchitis, rheumatism and scarlet fever, and is a good toner and dis-ease preventive.

Rosemary is a mint used for digestion, especially nervous indigestion. It helps in tension headaches, lowers high blood pressure and is a blood purifier and cleanser. The herb helps muscular pain, sciatica and neuralgia, and is used as a rinse to stop hair loss. An antidepressant (with scullcap), it eases tension, stimulates breast milk, prevents miscarriage and helps with menstrual cramps and PMS. Rosemary is also positive for colds and coughs, and is used as a wash or gargle for the mouth, gums and sore throats.

Scullcap is another member of the headache and migraine three: scullcap, hops and valerian. It's a major relaxant and stress reliever, used for insomnia, spasms and convulsions, hives, anxiety and nervous exhaustion. Use it as an antidepressant, and for help in overcoming cigarette, tranquilizer or alcohol addictions if it is used over a period of time. It is helpful in epilepsy, menstrual cramps, delayed menses and premenstrual syndrome. Use it also for rheumatism, gout, neuritis, muscle tremors or twitching, and for digestion and circulation.

Slippery Elm coats, relaxes, soothes and heals all tissues inside or out that it comes in contact with. Use it for diarrhea, colitis, gastritis, constipation, dysentery, food poisoning, diverticulitis, hiatal hernias, stomach cancer, sore throats, coughs, ulcers and hemorrhoids. In capsules with a lot of water, slippery elm stops vomiting and nausea. It is a douche for inflamed vaginal tissues. For debilitated women or children, slippery elm can be used as a highly digestible food. Use externally for boils, herpes, skin ulcers and eruptions, rashes and poison ivy. Drink lots of water with this herb.

Valerian is the natural basis for valium, but is without side effects. It is not a narcotic. It's the first herb to use for anxiety, stress, migraines, headaches or insomnia. Use it in epilepsy, pain relief, heart palpitations, muscle spasms and arthritis. For menstrual cramps try it with cramp bark; for tension and insomnia, try it with hops and/or scullcap. It is useful for women recovering from alcohol, and for children with measles or scarlet fever. Use it for shock, restlessness, any sort of pain or nervous debility. Billie Potts warns it can be habit forming, other sources say no. Do not overuse.

Violet is the holistic, nondrug treatment for all forms of cancer and is a cancer preventive. Use it with red clover for breast lumps, ovarian or uterine cysts, taken long term (see Red Clover) eight to sixteen ounces of infusion a day; eliminate caffeine. It is also used for bronchitis and upper respiratory congestion, rheumatism, cystitis, headaches and anxiety or stress. Use it externally as a wash for skin issues including skin cancer.

White Willow is the natural basis for aspirin. It relieves pain and reduces inflammation and fever without aspirin's side effects. Use it for arthritis, colds, flu, fevers, headaches, sore muscles, tonsillitis and pain. For tonsillitis, I made a mix with echinicea, comfrey, hyssop and white willow that was effective. It broke the fever, lessened inflammation and pain quickly and considerably. Use it for arthritis with burdock and alfalfa, and for colds with decongestant herbs like wintergreen.

Wintergreen is a strong tasting, strong scented herb for opening sinus congestions and colds. The taste is bad; use sparingly. The active ingredient in aspirin and white willow, salacin, is also present in wintergreen. The herb reduces fevers, inflammations and pain. Use it for rheumatism or arthritis attacks, for severe headaches and as a diuretic. It brings on menses and stimulates breast milk. Use externally in liniments and poultices for joint and muscular pain of lumbago, sciatica, rheumatism and arthritis.

Yarrow is a flu and fever herb, and also a blood purifier. It decreases menstrual flow and stops internal bleeding, aids amenorrhea, regulates the glands, liver and kidneys, helps bladder infections, balances blood circulation, helps respiratory dis-eases, stops diarrhea in infants, and lowers high blood pressure. For colds and flu, yarrow used generously at the beginning can stop it in twenty-four hours. Drink it warm for fevers. The tea is bitter but good tasting. Used externally, it is a douche for nonspecific vaginitis, a soak for hemorrhoids, and an antiseptic for rashes, cuts and wounds. Use it for children with measles or chicken pox internally and externally, and as a hair rinse. It helps in pleurisy, bleeding from the lungs, pneumonia, jaundice and hemorrhaging.

Yellow Dock is also a blood purifier, toner and cleanser. It is a lymphatic and liver cleanser and stimulant; it dissolves glandular tumors and is an anti-cancer agent. Use it for jaundice, hepatitis, gall bladder, liver congestion and anemia. Yellow dock is used for all skin problems, especially psoriasis and eruptions. It stops internal bleeding and heavy, excessive menstruation. A poultice heals cysts, burns, boils, sores and skin ulcers. Use it also for constipation and to move mucous through the kidneys.

Herbs work well with vitamins for healing, are internal cleansers and system regulators, have nutritional value and stimulate the body's immune system.[18] Use them along with prescription drugs if necessary, but in many cases herbs make doctors' visits and drugs unnecessary. Herbs help the body fight dis-ease by giving the immune system and energy a boost.

I would like to repeat that it is not necessary to use potions of a dozen different herbs. One to three is enough. Know what those herbs do and why you are using them. To quote my friend Rebecca Tallman, who asked that I stress this point:

> I really need to stress my standpoint on stacking herbs. I think it's just one more way of intimidating women into NOT taking control of their own health. Women usually turn to natural healing methods first out of a need to save money. Having less disposable income than men, we try whatever we can to control medical costs. Herbs are frequently difficult to find in the first place and when a woman discovers the cost of having (!) to buy several of them all at one time, she will abandon the whole idea as being more expensive than going to a doctor.
>
> If you use more than two-three herbs in one remedy, you are probably wasting your money by duplicating your effort. e.g., For relaxing and migraines, you don't need scullcap *and* hops *and* catnip *and* rosemary *and* valerian. For just relaxing use something mild—chamomile *or* hops *or* catnip, plus a bit of mint for flavor. For pain use scullcap first. If it isn't strong enough use valerian, but use it wisely—it's addictive. (That's where they get valium.)

I agree with this fully.

In the remedies that follow, where a number of herbs are suggested, look up what each does and pick the few that best fit your needs. If for menstrual issues you need an herb that balances cycles, one for pain and cramping, and one for PMS, try to find it all in one herb (raspberry, black cohosh or dong quai), or one that helps the hormone balance and another as a relaxant (raspberry and chamomile together). Don't duplicate, but choose the best fit and heed the warnings in the herb descriptions of when not to use a particular herb.

A great deal of alternative healing work is being done with **AIDS**, primarily looking for herbs, vitamins, homeopathics and diets that stimulate the immune system. A suggested mix of Chinese herbs includes, in Latin names, astragalus (yellow vetch) 20%, ligustrum (wax tree) 10%, schizandra 10%, eleuthero ginseng 15%, ganoderma 15%, white astractylodes 10%, codonopis 15% and licorice 5%. Garlic, echinacea and licorice are western herbs emphasized, also wheat grass, algae and anti-viral mushrooms.[19] Consider pau d'arco or violet with red clover.

For **arthritis**, I use alfalfa, burdock and white willow together. Also try comfrey, dandelion, dong quai, feverfew, garlic, licorice, valerian or wintergreen. Nettles, rosemary, sage, parsley, corn silk, black cohosh or cod liver oil taken daily are other suggestions.[20]

Garlic and/or cod liver oil are especially promising. Try feverfew for rheumatoid arthritis.

Bitter herbs are the key for **colds** and flu. Taking two capsules of equal amounts of cayenne with goldenseal every three hours with lots of water can stop or lessen a cold if started early enough. Boneset, yarrow or yellow dock are also positive, drunk hot. These are for the chilly type of colds. For colds with fever and heavy mucous, try rosehips, sorrel, comfrey, mint teas or raspberry leaf and vitamin C. If the cold becomes the flu, use boneset. Where there is hot, high fever and congestion, use elder flower and peppermint in a hot infusion, getting into bed to sweat it out.[21] Also suggested is garlic, and for congestion a mix of white willow, horehound or wintergreen, and hyssop. One herb store cold mix contains comfrey, echinacea, raspberry and licorice. For tonsillitis, gargle with goldenseal, a teaspoon to a pint of warm water.

For **cystitis** (recurrent bladder/urinary infections), drink a pint of unsweetened cranberry juice once an hour from the very first sign, and use vitamin C with calcium. This usually stops it within a few hours. Herbs include blue cohosh, boneset, buchu, burdock, coltsfoot, comfrey, damiana, dandelion, echinacea with yarrow, nettles, pau d'arco, raspberry leaf or yarrow. Billie Potts suggests uva ursi with echinacea if there is fever,[22] or echinacea with yarrow.

Dong quai or garlic/Kyolic perles have proved very positive for women with **high blood pressure**. Taken over a long period of time, monitoring pressure and doctors' medication doses, many women have been able to stop taking doctors' drugs. Other herbs to reduce high blood pressure are black cohosh, hyssop, motherwort, rosemary or yarrow. Raspberry leaf is suggested, as are passion flower, nettles or alfalfa.[23] For low blood pressure, garlic or dong quai are regulators; also try dandelion or licorice.

Licorice, garlic or dong quai are also suggested for **hypoglycemia** or any of the following herbs: alfalfa, cayenne, comfrey, dandelion, kelp, hawthorne or safflowers.[24] Since hypoglycemia and migraines often go together, try feverfew as a daily tea. Use herbs with vitamins; try pantothenic acid/B-5.

For **indigestion**, peppermint tea is the first thing to try, or rosemary, parsley, or peppermint with raspberry leaf. For nausea or vomiting, try slippery elm capsules, taken with enough water or warm tea. If you have food poisoning or early flu symptoms, it's more positive to get it all out. Take the slippery elm after vomiting to settle your stomach and prevent further vomiting. For gas, use peppermint, spearmint, comfrey, chamomile or alfalfa.[25] Herbs for morning sickness include alfalfa with peppermint, raspberry leaf or rosemary. Susun Weed suggests anise or fennel tea, raspberry leaf, peppermint, spearmint or ginger root tea.[26]

To heal **infections** with herbs, echinacea, hyssop, garlic, pau d'arco, yellow dock or goldenseal are all anti-viral, anti-microbial and anti-fungal. Recurrent colds, flus and tonsillitis respond well to garlic in the odorless Kyolic perles that may be used with echinacea. Comfrey and white willow are also positive. Use them with echinacea also. Goldenseal can be used internally or externally, as can comfrey, violet, yarrow, yellow dock or hops tincture.

For **menstrual** regulation, cramps and PMS, dong quai is a major herb, and black or blue cohosh are favorites of Native American women. Raspberry leaf with chamomile is especially positive, both for menstrual issues and in pregnancy. To lessen flows try comfrey, nettles, or goldenseal for hemorrhaging. Feverfew is positive for PMS, cramps and increasing flows, and pennyroyal or parsley increase flows and bring on menses. For premenstrual tension, try hops or scullcap with valerian for excessive pain. Nettles helps water retention, and motherwort or rosemary bring on menses, regulate cycles and prevent cramping. First to try here are raspberry leaf with chamomile, the cohoshes or dong quai. Do body-honoring affirmations.

Menopause issues respond to dong quai, black cohosh or licorice, also to motherwort, parsley or damiana. Some sources suggest ginseng, but dong quai is the women's ginseng and more positive. Shepherd's purse with alfalfa is positive for excessive pre-menopause menstrual hemorrhaging.[27] Licorice is a natural estrogen, as are motherwort or black cohosh root. For erratic cycles, heavy or clotted flows and hot flashes, Billie Potts suggests tincture of motherwort, two to four drops daily in water. Monitor heart rate and blood pressure carefully with this, as motherwort is a heart stimulant.[28] Licorice can also increase blood pressure. Parsley is a cycle regulator. Also remember vitamin E.

Women's **migraine** issues respond to a variety of herbs. Feverfew is promising but must be used daily over a long period of time, like dong quai. Try a tea of hops, scullcap and (occasionally) valerian, or hops, scullcap and catnip. Wintergreen, peppermint, nettles or white willow can help pain but are more for standard headaches than for migraines. In my experience, migraines are a combination of digestive issues, usually with hypoglycemia and emotional stress. Treating the hypoglycemia and learning to calm down will help the migraines, as well as keeping elimination regular. Try a sugar-free, chocolate-free and white flour-free diet, and eat several small meals a day of vegetables and whole grains.[29]

Practice meditation and relaxation techniques. My migraines stopped when I became a vegetarian and started using herbs—hops, scullcap and catnip. Use vitamins, especially B-complex. Billie Potts suggests a daily tea of scullcap, catnip and red clover.[30] (With catnip, you may have to fight your kittens for it!)

Multiple sclerosis is becoming a major healing issue for women, another immune system dis-ease, as are so many dis-eases of this century. Pau d'arco is promising, as is echinacea with garlic/Kyolic perles. Red clover is positive, possibly with yellow dock. Alfalfa is suggested as a nutrient and to help assimilate other herbs.[31] Velma Keith and Monteen Gordon suggest lobelia and relaxant herbs, plus vitamins,[32] but lobelia is under restriction (for no good reason) by the FDA. Lawrence Badgley in his book on AIDS suggests the same herbs and vitamins for MS as he does for AIDS, considering multiple sclerosis a viral dis-ease with an HIV-like virus as its source.[33] Correlations have been noted between high lead levels in the soil and water in areas of high incidence of multiple sclerosis and suggest that the dis-ease may be a form of environmental lead poisoning.[34] Much more work needs to be done with MS—it affects so many women and its incidence is increasing.

Osteoporosis, the thinning of bones in postmenopausal women, requires calcium and vitamin D. Herbs include alfalfa, with comfrey, dandelion or kelp.[35] Fluoridated water is implicated.

Herbs for the **skin** have a number of choices including aloe vera (aloes) with vitamin E externally, burdock, dandelion, pau d'arco, red clover, violet or yellow dock (externally and internally). Red clover and violet are used for all skin dis-eases including skin cancer. Pau d'arco is for psoriasis, burdock for all skin issues including acne. Velma Keith and Monteen Gordon suggest for acne: aloe vera, burdock, chaparral, dandelion, echinacea, kelp, clover, sarsaparilla or yellow dock. For eczema try aloe vera, burdock, comfrey, dandelion, echinacea, goldenseal or myrrh, and for psoriasis external aloe vera, burdock, dandelion, nettles or yellow dock internally.[36] A recipe for all skin disorders is two ounces clover, one ounce each of blue flag and burdock and one-half ounce of sassafras in a pint of cold water. Let stand overnight, then bring to a boil and simmer fifteen to twenty minutes. Cool, strain and drink an ounce and a half three times daily until the skin issue clears.[37]

Stress and insomnia are major women's issues and the cause of perhaps 85 percent of all dis-ease. The herbs for migraine are the herbs for stress, relaxant herbs to use with high protein, sugar-free, refined flour-free diets and meditation techniques. I use a mix of hops, scullcap and catnip, or replace the catnip with clover or feverfew. Ginseng is suggested for stress, but is a stimulant and less positive for women than dong quai. For immune system depression caused by stress, try garlic perles. Feverfew, hops, scullcap or black cohosh are stress reducers, also chamomile, raspberry, rosehips or rosemary. Use alfalfa for its nutrients and assimilation properties, along with other choices. For insomnia, hops is the classic herb.

For **vaginal infections**, blue cohosh, comfrey or raspberry leaf are positive taken internally. Try equal parts of goldenseal, myrrh and echinacea in size 00 capsules, taking two capsules three times a day for six weeks. As a douche, use goldenseal with myrrh for vaginitis and yeast infections, or garlic or comfrey as douches, and slippery elm as a douche for inflamed vaginal tissues. Yarrow or calendula are helpful as douches for nonspecific vaginitis. For yeast infections and candida albicans (recurrent or systemic yeast) pau d'arco or daily garlic perles have proved positive and garlic with bayberry bark douches. Try acidophilus bacillus internally and as a douche. Yarrow, sage or comfrey teas used as a douche are also positive for yeast infections, and blue cohosh as a douche and tea for vaginal discharges.[38] Oatstraw tea as a drink and a douche is suggested.[39] For ovarian, uterine or breast **cysts** try red clover with violet, a pint a day over six months to dissolve them. Dong quai is also positive. Echinacea is helpful for pelvic inflammation or mastitis. When yeast is a problem, avoid eating sugar; it activates the organisms.

These are only a few of the women's dis-eases that herbs help heal. One chapter cannot begin to cover herbalism, either in types of herbs or healing issues, and Chinese herbs have barely been touched here. Read the books suggested and referenced in this chapter and work with herbs in order to go further. Talk with other women and share experiences and information. Women usually don't believe how well herbs work until they have tried them. Herbs work more slowly than drugs but more thoroughly and without side effects. When using them for acute issues, continue dosing for a few days after symptoms disappear, then decrease slowly to prevent recurrence. when using them for chronic issues, herbs must be used daily over a period of several months.

I would like to thank Billie Potts for her powerful and important women's herbal *Witches Heal*, and express my delight that it has finally been reprinted. I would also like to thank Rebecca Tallman for her sane and informed input to this chapter, and for her herb suggestions and recipes.

NOTES

1. Ted Kaptchuk, *The Web That Has No Weaver*, (New York, Congdon and Weed, Inc., 1983), pp. 81–83.

2. Judy Chicago, *The Dinner Party: A Symbol of Our Heritage*, (New York, Doubleday Books, 1979), pp.116–119.

3. *Ibid.*, p. 123.

4. *Ibid.*, pp. 127–130.

5. Barbara Ehrenreich and Dierdre English, *For Her Own Good, 150 Years of the Experts' Advice to Women*, (New York, Anchor Books, 1979), pp.36–37.

6. Judy Chicago, *The Dinner Party*, pp. 148–150.

7. Barbara Ehrenreich and Dierdre English, *For Her Own Good*, pp. 36–37.

8. Billie Potts, *Witches Heal: Lesbian Herbal Self-Sufficiency*, (Bearsville, NY, Hecuba's Daughters Press, 1981), p. 9. This wonderful book is now back in print from Du Reve Publications, POB 7772, Ann Arbor, MI 48107. Highly recommended.

9. *Ibid.*, p. 10.

10. *Ibid.*, P. 11.

11. David Hoffman, *The Holistic Herbal*, (Scotland, The Findhorn Press, 1983), pp. 150–151.

12. Billie Potts, *Witches Heal*, p. 15.

13. *Ibid.*, pp. 13–14.

14. David Hoffman, *The Holistic Herbal*, p. 154.

15. *Ibid.*, p. 153.

16. *Ibid.*, p. 137 ff. Also John Meyer, *The Herbalist*, (Glenwood, IL, Meyerbooks, 1918), p. 148 ff.

17. Kathi Keville, "Strengthening Your Immune System with Herbs," handout reprint from *Vegetarian Times*, July, 1985.

18. Velma Keith and Monteen Gordon, *The How To Herb Book*, pp. 1–2.

19. Lawrence Badgley, MD, *Healing AIDS Naturally*, (San Bruno, CA, Human Energy Press, 1987), pp. 166–204.

20. Mildred Jackson, ND and Terri Teague, ND, DC, *The Handbook of Alternatives to Chemical Medicine*, (Berkeley, CA, Bookpeople, 1975), pp. 16–17.

21. Billie Potts, *Witches Heal*, pp. 107–109.

22. *Ibid.*, p. 138.

23. Mildred Jackson and Terri Teague, *The Handbook of Alternatives to Chemical Medicine*, p. 88.

24. Velma Keith and Monteen Gordon, *The How To Herb Book*, (Pleasant Grove, VT, Mayfield Publishing, 1984) , p. 213.

25. *Ibid.*, p. 205.

26. Susun Weed, *WiseWoman Herbal for the Childbearing Year*, (Woodstock, NY, Ash Tree Publishing, 1985), pp. 24–25.

27. Billie Potts, *Witches Heal*, pp. 132–133.

28. *Ibid.*

29. Mildred Jackson and Terri Teague, *Handbook of Alternatives to Chemical Medicine*, p. 81.

30. Billie Potts, *Witches Heal*, p. 110.

31. Mildred Jackson and Terri Teague, *Handbook of Alternatives to Chemical Medicine*, p. 32.

32. Velma Keith and Monteen Gordon, *The How To Herb Book*, pp. 218–219.

33. Lawrence Badgley, MD, *Healing AIDS Naturally*, p. 7.

34. Prevention Magazine Staff, *The Complete Book of Minerals*, (Emmaus, PA, Rodale Press, 1972), pp. 455–461.

35. Velma Keith and Monteen Gordon, *The How To Herb Book*, p. 221.

36. *Ibid.*, pp. 189, 203, 224.

37. Mildred Jackson and Terri Teague, *Handbook of Alternatives to Chemical Medicine*, p. 105.

38. Cobra, "Herbcraft: Remedies for Vaginitis," in *Goddess Rising*, (4006 First St. NE, Seattle, WA 98105), Issue #20, Spring, 1988.

39. Mildred Jackson and Terri Teague, *Handbook of Alternatives to Chemical Medicine*, p. 71.

Chapter Nine

—————————○—————————

Homeopathy

Though developed two hundred years ago by a man, homeopathy has origins in matriarchies and has been used and researched extensively by women. The system would not have survived its early (and continuing) assaults from the American Medical Association and the western medical establishment were it not for the persistence and work of its women practitioners. Homeopathy is one of the few modern medical systems that has shown consistent equality to women, though male writings—often sexist and racist—need rewriting. Based partly on women's herbalism, but different from it in many ways, homeopathy is a system used extensively with standard medicine in Europe, South America and India, and is surviving repression in the United States. There are a large percentage of women practitioners of homeopathy, including some women MDs.

For most acute dis-eases homeopathy can effectively be practiced at home, but for chronic issues the skill is complex and requires extensive training and experience. The National Center for Homeopathy defines it as "a postgraduate holistic medical specialty."[1] Formally trained homeopaths are taught in homeopathic colleges, and in England and India homeopathic doctors are as popular or more popular than allopathic ones. In the United States despite official rejection by the medical community and restricted training, there are an increasing number of homeopathic physicians, many of them holistically oriented women. Many more women homeopaths are not doctors but are nurses, chiropractors, naturopaths, etc. Though the National Center would like homeopathy to be accepted by the AMA, in the United States it remains a wholistic healing method with at least partial emphasis on self-help. This chapter is an introduction to homeopathy. It is perhaps the most complex of the healing systems discussed in this book.

The concept of *similia similibus curentur*, 'like cures like,' is the basis of homeopathic theory, and the word 'homeopathy' means 'like suffering.' The idea of a cure based on the use of an herb, mineral, metal or bacteria that causes the sick woman's dis-ease symptoms when given to a healthy woman, is an idea going back to the matriarchies. To apply 'like cures like,' if a woman shows symptoms that resemble lead poisoning, a highly diluted homeopathic remedy of lead can be expected to cure her symptoms. The remedy is so dilute that probably no actual molecule of lead, only the vibratory aura essence left by the succussion process, remains in it. The dis-ease-causing substance in highly dilute form stimulates the woman's immune system to reject and heal the dis-ease.

Long ago the Delphic Oracle pronounced, " That which makes sick shall heal."[2] Delphi was an ancient women's and Goddess center for healing and prophecy existing up to the fifth century BCE, dedicated to Gaia the Earth Mother. In the patriarchal takeover, Delphi became Apollo's temple, but its roots are female and matriarchal. Hippocrates in the fourth century BCE referred to the law of similars, and he probably got the idea from matriarchal tradition. At the very least, he would have been aware of Delphi. Paracelsus, the fifteenth century rebel who is credited with starting western medicine (but didn't, remember Hildegard of Bingen), admitted that he had learned his healing from witches. He was a proponent of the 'like cures like' theory. Paracelsus is also the discoverer (I will not say inventor) of the doctrine of signatures that is used in gemstone healing. The idea there is that what a stone or herb resembles is what it may be used for. A yellow stone such as citrine, or a yellow herb like yellow dock, can be used for gallbladder and bile issues, since bile is a yellow fluid in the body. This is another form of 'like cures like.' The law of similars was known in China, Greece, South America, Native America and Asia in early times.[3]

Homeopathy as it's known today was developed by Samuel Hahnemann (1755-1843), a noted German physician, chemist and writer who gave up standard/allopathic medicine because he felt he was doing more harm than good with it. Working for a living mostly as a medical translator, he disagreed with a book he was translating (Cullen's *Materia Medica*) on the actions and effects of chinchona (quinine), the Peruvian Bark used as an anti-malarial for intermittent fevers. Taking the herb himself, he discovered that the symptoms the bark was supposed to cure were the symptoms he developed from taking it. After using chinchona to cure a woman of intermittent fevers that resembled what he had experienced on taking the herb, he began to research further.

For the next twenty years Hahnemann tested various herbs and drugs (they were usually the same in this era before synthesized medicines) one at a time for what they would do when given to a healthy person. He controlled these 'provings' carefully. What the drug manifested in a healthy woman proved to be the illness it would cure in a dis-ease state. He first wrote about his findings in 1796 in a respected German medical journal and published his *Organon de Rationellen Heilkunde*, (*The Classification of Practical Medicine*), with his full findings in 1810. His materia medica of provings was expanded and revised several times before his death.[4] Though Edward Jenner discovered smallpox vaccine in 1798 by a similar theory, using small diluted amounts of the dis-ease agent to immunize with, Jenner was embraced by the medical establishment, but Hahnemann was not. He was arrested in 1820 for dispensing his own medicines and hounded out of Leipzig.[5] This split between methods has become the split between standard medicine and homeopathy.

On testing and administering his first medicines, Hahnemann discovered serious side effects. He could not use the dis-ease-causing/dis-ease-curing agents full strength without toxic symptoms, and worked to find out how dilute a dose would still be effective to heal the dis-ease it matched. The process of potentization he developed is unique to homeopathy and a contrast to the medical system's overdosing of drugs and medicines and its disregard of side effects. Less is more in homeopathic remedies—the more dilute the remedy the more potent it's considered to be. Potentization begins usually with an herbal tincture, and one drop of the tincture is diluted in ninety-nine drops of alcohol or water. This is then pounded by succussion, shaking it vigorously or striking it against a firm surface. One drop of the diluted, succussed mixture is then diluted again in ninety-nine drops of alcohol or water and again succussed, and the process is repeated a number of times. Remedies diluted one drop of tincture to ninety-nine of alcohol are called centesimal potencies and are labeled with a c, as 6c, 12c, 30c, 200c, 1000c, 10,000c, 50,000c or 100,000c, depending on the number of times the process is repeated. Remedies diluted one drop of tincture to ten drops of alcohol are called decimal potencies and labeled with an x, as 6x, 12x, 30x, 200x, etc. Centesimal potencies sometimes use just the number, without the c; decimal potencies (of much less strength) are always marked with the x.[6]

A dilution of fifteen times or less (15x, 15c or lower) is

considered a lower potency, and some homeopaths use these exclusively. The more dilute the potency, the more powerful and long lasting it is, though the actual amount of the original herb or substance lessens with each dilution. Beyond a dilution of 24x or 12c there may not be any molecules remaining of the original tincture, yet each dilution and succussion makes the remedy more potent. Higher potencies last longer but run risks of greater aggravations, healing crises in which the woman's symptoms get worse before they get better. Aggravations are considered positive, and indicate the right choice of remedy, but some cases should be handled by experienced homeopaths. Depending on the practitioner, most homeopaths choose low potencies for chronic issues and high ones for acute dis-eases. For women beginning homeopathy, potencies of 6x to 30c are recommended for treating acute illnesses at home.

The idea of such infinitesimal doses is strange to western women, who are raised with the idea that if a little works, more must be better. This is pretty much the attitude of the medical establishment, that uses drugs in too high doses and with too many side effects, some of them fatal. To understand why such small doses work, return to the idea of woman's aura as her life force energy field that determines her state of health. A homeopathic remedy, devoid by dilution of probably any of the original tincture because of succussion, retains the energy pattern of the tincture herb or substance. The highly energized dilution becomes energy itself affecting women's unseen aura bodies that are also comprised of energy. Where in using herbs and vitamins women are doing physical level healing, homeopathy returns to a method that involves the ki and aura bodies.

The diluted remedy is placed on tiny beads of milk sugar and taken under the tongue, or can be given in a liquid. A high potency remedy might be taken only once, as the dosage is not repeated as long as the changes it initiates continue. Lower potency doses in acute healing issues are repeated more often, three or four times a day or even as often as every few minutes until the symptoms start to change. Once healing begins, the dose is not repeated until the changes stop. A woman telling me about her experiences with homeopathy gave her child, who had been exposed to scarlet fever and was breaking out in a rash, a homeopathic dose of belladonna 6c. She used a dose every hour until the symptoms changed, and the potentially dangerous dis-ease was totally gone by the next day. Potencies of 6x to 30c are the recommended dosage to use for home healing of acute issues such as this one.[7] Because the dose is so small, there are no side effects other than the possible and usually short aggravation of symptoms. The more likely risk is that the remedy won't work if it's the wrong one. Dosage is less critical than choosing the right remedy.

The complexity of finding the right remedy is what makes homeopathy so challenging. Each drug proving, the testing of a substance on a healthy individual, develops a series of highly specific symptoms for each remedy, called its drug picture. The homeopath taking a case study finds the remedy that closest fits the individual woman's symptoms, matching her symptom picture to the closest drug picture. Since even in simple dis-eases no two women's symptoms are exactly alike, and since there are a total of 2000–3000 drug pictures in the full homeopathic materia medica, choosing the precisely correct remedy is seldom simple. Not all of each remedy's multitude of symptoms is operative in a specific dis-ease, either.

A great deal of research and study goes into choosing the best remedy, and if in acute issues no change in symptoms has occurred in twenty-four hours, the process has to start all over again, as the right remedy is yet to be found. The choice is based entirely on symptoms, rather than dis-ease names or labels. There is a definite right and wrong in homeopathy; a remedy either works or doesn't. Only one remedy is taken at a time in classical homeopathy, to be able to follow the changes and what caused them.

To do a homeopathic healing, a woman is questioned in extreme detail about her symptoms. If it's a headache, she is questioned about where it hurts, what the pain feels like, whether she is hot or cold, what makes her feel better or worse, what time of day it develops, what she wants to eat or not eat, and more. She is asked about her emotional and mental symptoms as much as about physical ones, and these are as important, or more so, than physical aspects of her dis-ease. A homeopathic casetaking can take an hour or more for an involved chronic issue, but less for simpler acute ones. At the easiest and clearest, the process is still thorough. Then the homeopath goes to a repertory, an index of symptoms, looking up every possible remedy listed for each of the woman's symptoms in a materia medica, a book of remedy descriptions. (An experienced practitioner may know enough so that she will not need to look it up.) She seeks the remedy that includes all of the major symptoms and as many of the lesser ones as possible, and that closely fits the emotional state. Reading the possible drug pictures/descriptions, she chooses the one that most closely describes that particular headache. When the right remedy is chosen and used, results are rapid and often amazing. Homeopathy is highly successful, often healing ills beyond the range of standard medicine.

The complete materia medica with repertory (several versions by different editors are available) is a book of 1100 pages or more in very small print, costing about twenty dollars. Computers have entered homeopathy, but the comparison and choices are still up to the individual healer and the process of choosing a remedy from so much information is painstaking. The remedies themselves, found at herb stores and food co-ops, or at the several homeopathic pharmacies for order by mail, are relatively cheap, running three to five dollars for a vial or bottle. Kits are available containing several frequently used remedies from about fifteen dollars, and I recommend a thirty remedy kit if you can afford it. Women can also make their own. Compared to medicine, homeopathy is affordable, and when it works it works very well.

When it doesn't work, the reason is usually the wrong choice of remedy, the remedy being rendered inert before taking it, or the antidoting of the remedy by a strong fragrance in the woman's environment. A remedy needs to be handled with great care to retain potency, especially since you can't tell by looking at it if it's 'good' or not. Exposing a remedy to direct sunlight, great heat, odors, or contaminating it by touching or dropping it can make the remedy or dose ineffective. Strong odors such as peppermint or camphor can discontinue the healing process, also drinking coffee, mint tea or fennel tea, severe emotional trauma, dental work or applying camphorated products to the skin (sunbreeze, tiger balm, etc.). Women using homeopathic remedies avoid these influences for the time of using the remedy. Caffeine and peppermint toothpastes are big offenders here, but non-peppermint toothpastes are available at healthfood stores and decaffeinated coffee may or may not interfere.

The healing process in homeopathy has prescribed patterns for occurrence, as explained by Hering's Law of Cure which has three parts. The first is that a woman's body moves to dislodge disease from internal to external levels. A skin issue is less serious than a heart issue, and an external dis-ease is easier to heal. When finding and using the right remedy picture, the woman may experience a change in her symptoms, as the symptoms move from internal to more external levels. If psychological symptoms lessen but physical ones temporarily increase, the remedy is working. Mental and emotional levels are considered to be deeper than physical levels. A woman with asthma may develop a skin rash as the dis-ease moves outward, but the rash clears as her healing continues and her lungs clear first. Standard medicine would treat the rash with cortisone, sending the dis-ease inward again, and reactivating the asthma. Homeopathy classically traces asthma to a child's suppressed skin rash or eczema.

The second part of Hering's Law is that healing proceeds from upper to lower parts of the body. The healing is occurring if pain in an arthritic woman's neck has decreased, though her hands still hurt. Shoulder joints see improvement before knees. If a woman with sick headaches finds that her head hurts less, though her stomach remains upset, the healing is started. Cures that start in upper body parts move downward. Her headaches become less, and then the upset stomachs follow.

Hering's third law is that symptoms disappear in the reverse order of their appearance. Newest symptoms disappear first, and sometimes the woman re-experiences an old symptom that she hasn't had in a while. The return of an old symptom usually happens when doctors' synthetic drugs have suppressed it, as in the skin rash of asthma, and this occurrence is seen as positive. Where medicine suppresses symptoms, homeopathy releases them from the aura. Reactions of this sort, or aggravations, don't last long and, when they leave, the woman sees positive and definite differences in her well-being. It is important to let these recurrences and aggravations happen and run their course, not to suppress them with medications.[8] Other forms of women's healing see these healing crises and patterns of healing, and recognize them as releasing the layers of the dis-ease.

Homeopathy is a method of aura healing, positive for most diseases, but it has some limits. When there is a broken bone, it requires standard medical attention, though homeopathic remedies are helpful to ease pain, prevent shock, and calm the woman emotionally. Homeopathy treats body, emotions, mind and spirit, rather than the body only, but some physical level issues require physical level healing responses. That the system treats the four bodies helps make it a women's healing method, and part of its reason for success. Less than a hundred years ago, many physicians and surgeons in the United States were also homeopaths, and they used both allopathic and homeopathic methods together. This is still true in England, France and in a number of other countries. Homeopathy can prevent the need for many surgeries and for many toxic chemical drugs with their attendant side effects, but at very grave times homeopathy is not enough. Other limits of homeopathy are listed below.[9]

1. Homeopathy is not indicated by itself in a life-threatening

situation when speed is a life-or-death matter: a heart attack or obstruction of breathing in asthma or broken bones. Do what works fastest using homeopathy as a backup.

2. Remedies may be ineffective when nutrition or lifestyle issues are the cause of the dis-ease. If a woman is deficient in vitamin B-12 because she has been a strict vegetarian for several years, she needs B-12 and not a homeopathic remedy. If a woman's dis-ease is from her environment, if she is getting sick because she lives in a neighborhood too highly polluted for her body's tolerance, homeopathics might make her more comfortable, but her cure depends on her moving to a more positive place.

3. It can take a long time by trial and error to find the right homeopathic remedy, especially in chronic dis-eases, and if the woman is uncomfortable, she may want to seek other healing methods first, or along with homeopathy. Homeopathy can work along with doctors' drugs, but this is not optimal.

4. A long-term dis-ease becomes incurable after a certain point, and after that homeopathy can help the woman to greater comfort but cannot cure her.

5. If a woman takes a homeopathic that is not the right remedy for her, she may eventually experience the symptoms that remedy is meant to cure. To prevent this, it is recommended not to take remedies for acute issues longer than a week without response. If a remedy has not had a healing effect within twenty-four hours in most acute cases, it is probably the wrong remedy.

The limitations of homeopathy are similar to those for other forms of women's healing. Reiki, for example, is used for accidents but along with standard medical techniques, as are other forms of healing. Common sense says that when you are uncomfortable to seek healing in the most positive way, which may be homeopathy or not. A woman with appendicitis can try a remedy, herbs, vitamins or bodywork, but if her appendix is about to burst she needs surgery. Use alternative healing methods afterwards to help her recover. When environment is the cause, no healing method takes the place of eliminating a negative variable. I have counselled a number of women with migraines to find a less stressful job or learn to defuse their stress issues, so that the variety of healing methods for migraines is no longer needed. In the case of wrong remedies, the wrong homeopathic treatment may change the woman's symptoms, but it usually just won't work.

Women healers are also aware that dis-eases can reach a point of no return, and they are aware of the cycle of life and death. If a woman's dis-ease is permanent, help her to live with it in the easiest ways possible. If a woman is dying, help her to be comfortable—physically, emotionally, mentally and spiritually. Goddess women and witches accept the turning Wheel and the laws of karma. Medical heroics with respirators and heart transplants may hold off physical death for awhile, but they ignore the qualities of what life really is. The Karen Ann Quinlan case was a tragedy. If a woman has chosen to pass over, don't try to prevent or stop her and don't deny the facts. Her work on this plane, for this lifetime, is done. The healer's part in this is to respect and ease the process in whatever ways she can.

Homeopathy has some obvious differences from standard allopathic medicine, but because it administers remedies that may be seen as drugs it has some similarities to it, too. Allopathic medicine uses synthetic drugs in doses as large as the woman's body can tolerate (and sometimes more); homeopathy uses natural tinctures diluted to the lowest possible dose via the process of succussion and potentization. Patriarchal medicine treats the physical body only, while homeopathy treats the whole woman, body, emotions, mind and spirit in a very individualized way. The medical system sees patients at a rate of six or so an hour, prescribing synthetic drugs that run from ten to hundreds of dollars a month, but always prescribing one or several drugs. Homeopathy casetakings can require several hours and can admittedly be expensive, but the homeopath recommends a single remedy very carefully and remedies are included in office visits. She may give one dose of a remedy and repeat it at intervals, or not repeat it for several months. The treatment and follow-up are highly personalized, where allopathic medicine is more and more computerized and high-tech. The slogan in homeopathy is "the patient, not the cure." In many issues, self-help is possible and encouraged with homeopathy, as compared to the doctor-is-god mystique of modern male medicine.

It's interesting to know the American history of homeopathy and the AMA. The politics are typical of male medicine mirroring the ways the medical system has repressed and destroyed women's healing. By 1800, the witch burnings were over and the male medical profession in Europe and the United States was for the most part established. Herbalism was being replaced by drugs, soon to be synthetic chemical drugs, of the more-is-better philosophy. The openly practicing woman healer was gone, but there were still herb women and midwives, especially away from the cities. These women were discredited as 'dirty and ignorant,' since they were in competition to organized medicine, and homeopathy was attacked for the same reason, but in different ways.

The herbal healers had the state-of-the-art medical knowledge of their time until they died in the witch burnings. Homeopathy carried herbalism further, making it into a scientific study, but the new medical profession disliked it. It used low cost, nontoxic herbal preparations that could not be patented or sold at high prices by the beginning drug industry, and homeopathic doctors often made their own remedies. Unlike the women healers, however, homeopaths were male medical school graduates and less easy to dismiss or get rid of. Their methods were more civilized than the early medical system's, and like the witch-midwives they took business away from standard doctors because of their greater effectiveness.

> In 1900 a comparison of mortality rates among homeopathic and conventional medical patients throughout the United States and Europe showed that between two and eight times as many homeopathic patients with life-threatening infectious diseases survived as compared with those receiving conventional medical care of the day.[10]

The first medical society in the United States was the American Institute of Homeopathy, begun in 1844 when homeopathy was a rapidly growing field. By 1900, twenty to twenty-five percent of American doctors practicing in cities were homeopaths, with over a hundred homeopathic hospitals and twenty-two homeopathic medical schools.[11] A doctor's association for standard practitioners formed their own medical society in 1846—the American Medical Association—almost solely for the purpose of fighting homeopathy.

This early AMA conducted a purge of medical societies, expelling all non-standard (homeopathic) physicians. In 1855, they declared that any physician who consulted or referred patients to a homeopath would be expelled from the society, which meant they would be expelled from practicing medicine. They sought and won legislation to support their goals. Homeopathic practice and training were highly restricted, and homeopathy became synonymous with quackery. Homeopathy declined—because it couldn't withstand the onslaught, because of infighting, and because new medical drugs (antibiotics) worked more quickly and seemingly miraculously, overshadowing homeopathy's slower and more thorough ways.[12]

Homeopathy survived because of women's support and practice. The first women's medical college in the world was a homeopathic college, the Boston Female Medical College, started in 1848. It merged with Boston University in 1873, which was also a homeopathic college. Women were welcomed into the American Institute of Homeopathy by 1871 but were refused by the AMA until 1915 and then only admitted in very small numbers. The allopathic medical schools are still slow to accept women students.[13] Homeopathy was popular among all classes of women, poor and rich, but particularly among the educated and upper classes. The press supported homeopathy, and homeopathic medical schools were equal to or better than standard ones. Yet, the AMA was effective in suppressing homeopathy, as it had suppressed women healers and midwives. The acceptance of women by homeopathy was only another reason to destroy it, but some lay practitioners continued.

> By 1950, all the homeopathic colleges in the United States were either closed or no longer teaching homeopathy. There were only 50 to 150 practicing homeopathic physicians, and most of these were over 50 years old.[14]

Homeopathy is reemerging, due to the return of holistic healing and due to its strong popularity and proven effectiveness in England, Holland, Asia, South America and India. There are over 120 homeopathic medical schools in India alone, and homeopathy in other countries is on a par with allopathic medicine. Seventy percent of those who try it in England are pleased with it,[15] a far higher rate of satisfaction than standard medicine gets. Homeopathy is not dead, and Goddess women's healing is very much alive, and the two seem ready to meet. The number of women practitioners of homeopathy is increasing.

Homeopathy for acute dis-eases, dis-eases that are self-limiting as in flus, colds and accidents—plus women's issues where it is positive to stay away from doctors for as long as possible—are self-healing issues. Dis-eases that are chronic and not self-limiting are harder to find the correct remedy for and require some help from an experienced woman homeopath or homeopathic MD. The more practice and success a woman has healing acute conditions, the more effective she becomes for difficult ones, so it is better to start with clear-cut dis-eases, moving toward harder issues. Any woman can gain that expertise by choice and practice, and as the *I Ching* says, 'perseverance furthers.'

In the healing information that follows, the woman goes to a homeopathic materia medica to compare the suggested remedy picture with her own symptoms. If several remedies are suggested, she checks each to find which closest fits her own dis-ease. A materia medica and repertory is suggested for women wishing to do homeopathy in a bigger way, but many of the homeopathy healing guides contain smaller materia medicas. No two women's healing issues are alike, no matter how simple. Since homeopathy is designed to work for specific symptoms in great detail, the remedies to choose are very precise. Take the suggested remedy in low potency, about 6x to 30c dosage, every one to six hours, depending on severity. If there is no improvement overnight, the choice is probably not the right one. (Changes usually occur within an hour, often less.) Read the remedy picture in a materia medica for other choices.

If the remedy is ineffective, check also to see if something in the environment is antidoting it. If you drink coffee, stop for the length of the healing. Any strong smelling odor—camphor, mint or menthol, as well as fragrant herb oils—can render a remedy inert. Chest rubs, eucalyptus cough drops, tiger balm or dental work can be antidotes. If antidoting happens, stop the problem substance and continue taking the remedy. If, in using the remedy, symptoms get better, then return, repeat the remedy; if the symptoms change, check the remedy descriptions, as a different one may be needed.[16] As long as the remedy is working and symptoms improve, no more doses are taken. Avoid touching the tiny pellets when putting them under your tongue, spill them into and out of the bottle cap. Avoid eating for half an hour or drinking liquids for fifteen minutes after taking a remedy. Homeopathy is also useful for animals.

Alternative healing methods of every sort are being explored as healing for **AIDS/ARC**. The politics of the dis-ease are horrific, along with the dis-ease itself, and attempts are being made to find a virus that is probably an aftereffect, rather than a cause. AIDS has been with us for many years under a variety of other names, but the medical system refuses to consider the environment as its source and as the source of all the other immune system break-down dis-eases. AIDS is not alone, but is in a class with such ills as arthritis, multiple sclerosis, hepatitis, lupus, Epstein-Barr Syndrome, herpes, allergies, asthma and candida albicans. When a real look for causes is finally done, my opinion is that it will point to some poison in the environment—toxicities in the water, air, soil or food supply that the government has chosen to allow. Lead is already being implicated in multiple sclerosis. Homeopaths credit the increase in immune system dis-eases to the use of vaccinations, steroids and antibiotics, and some believe that reaction to smallpox vaccine may trigger AIDS.[17] Another factor is inherited predisposition, compounded by contracting recurrent sexually transmitted dis-eases (STDs) and suppressing them with drugs. The body's immune system can't operate in a toxic environment, or in one where symptoms are repressed instead of healed.

In the meantime, alternative healers are working extensively with AIDS and other immune deficiency dis-eases. Medical establishment drugs for AIDS have horrible side effects, while natural healing methods have none and are non-toxic. Herbs, vitamins and nutrition are some of the methods being explored. In homeopathy, a substance that causes a dis-ease in healthy people is potentized by dilution and succussion to create the remedy for that dis-ease. One homeopathic remedy made in this way that's being tried is cyclosporin.[18] Cyclosporin is the drug used to suppress organ rejection in transplant patients, and persons with AIDS/ARC experience the same immune system depression that cyclosporin intentionally creates. Potentized cyclosporin is being tried, with positive results, by homeopathic physicians.

Another homeopathic remedy being used for AIDS is the potentized and succussed dilution of killed typhoid virus, a nosode called Typhoidinum. A homeopathic remedy made from a microbe is called a nosode and various ones are homeopathic mainstays. In exploring the symptoms of typhoid, AIDS researcher Lawrence Badgley discovered that the symptoms are the same as those for AIDS, with the difference that in typhoid it happens very quickly from start to finish, and in AIDS the dis-ease process occurs over much more time. He is having success with these remedies, and suggests further remedy pictures for the dis-ease.[19] In these cases, seek the help of a homeopathic physican—do not try to self-treat. Homeopathic remedies are given in the latin names, their herb names end this chapter.

For **colds and flu**, there are a number of remedies. Again look for the one that best fits the woman needing it. Check the full remedy pictures in a materia medica. Aconite may be the homeopathic to use at first in a cold (also in cystitis) of sudden onset, after exposure to dry winds. Arsenicum colds are characterized by running noses with discharge that burns the upper lip and by sneezing after weather changes. Nux vomica colds begin with a woman who is chilly, who has a feeling of irritation high inside her nose. If the cold starts with a feeling of rawness in the throat and a cough, try Causticum. If it's a sticking sensation in the throat and a dry cough at the beginning of a cold, try Hepar sulph, and especially if the woman is prone to bronchitis. If the cold is a chest cold, try Ferrum phos. For viral colds, try Gelsemium or Bryonia.[20]

Belladonna colds include high fevers and dry flushed faces. In an early, acute respiratory infection/cold with undefined symptoms, try Belladonna first, and then Ferrum phos. If there is a heavy nasal discharge the remedy may be Natrum mur. Arsenicum and Bryonia are for colds with coughs; spongia for a croupy cough. For a cold with cough and sore throat, congestion and hoarseness, try Rhus tox.[21] The repertory of cold symptoms and the homeopathic possibilities for them run several pages long.

Most of these remedies are positive for flu symptoms as well, but Gelsemium seems to be the first flu remedy to reference. Symptoms include fever and chills, little thirst, runny nose and raw throat, sometimes headaches, and weakness, tiredness and a wish to be left alone. Symptoms for Bryonia flus are characterized by irritability and reluctance to move because it hurts. In a Rhus tox flu, there are stiff achy muscles, and in a Eupatorium perfoliatum flu, the woman has deeper aches and pains, a dry hacking cough, and sudden onset of nasal discharge with sneezing at the beginning.[22] Oscillococcinum is a remedy considered to be eighty to ninety percent effective for flu when taken within forty-eight hours of onset.[23] If the symptom is a simple fever, try Belladonna or Aconite. Again, go to a homeopathic materia medica or treatment guide to compare the symptoms and pick the remedy closest to your own dis-ease.

Cystitis in women is treated homeopathically by several remedy choices, the first being Causticum, which can also be used as a preventive. Where there are urinary or kidney stones, Berberis is positive, and Margery Blackie—the Queen of England's personal physician—says it can prevent surgeries.[24] Cantharis is also suggested as primary, for burning and irritation of the urinary tract, and Sarsaparilla, Mercurius, Nux vomica, Pulsatilla or Apis.[25] In Cantharis, there is urging but little urination. Sarsaparilla is used when urethral pain is worst at the end of urinating, and Mercurius is indicated when the symptoms are worst at night. Nux vomica cystitis has burning or pressing pain during urination, urethral pain that is needlelike. It is used when the attacks occur after alcohol, coffee or medication use. Apis for cystitis is used in severe pain, strong urging with little urine flow, and an abdomen sensitive to touch.[26]

For **indigestion** with severe vomiting, nausea, diarrhea and stomach pain, try Arsenicum. The woman with this remedy picture is thirsty and has chills; she fears her illness and even fears she might die of it. If Arsenicum fails, try Phosphorus, especially when the woman is unable to keep water down, but vomits it up and has a general feeling of emptiness and weakness inside. When indigestion is marked by cramping abdominal pains, especially after anger, that are relieved by pressure and warmth, Colocynthis is the remedy, also for infants' colic. If she seeks more warmth and less pressure, try Magnesia phos. If the dis-ease occurs suddenly,

Belladonna may help in early stages—the woman or child has a fever, a red flushed face, and she feels dull.

Bryonia is the remedy for severe gastritis with nausea, vomiting and abdominal pain all worsened by motion. When digestion is upset from overeating, emotional issues, alcohol, coffee or medications, try Nux vomica. Pulsatilla may help women whose indigestion comes from rich foods, or less severe and ordinary indigestion. Nausea alone, with clean tongue and no relief from vomiting, responds to Ipecac. When profuse yellow diarrhea is the main symptom, try Podophyllum; for violent, exhausting diarrhea, try Veratrum album. For motion sickness, try Cocculus or Petroleum; Cocculus is the remedy for severe motion sickness that makes the woman need to lie down, and worsens with cold or the smell of food. Petroleum is for motion sickness where the woman becomes faint or pale, breaking out in a cold sweat.[27] Constipation responds to Bryonia, Nux vomica, Opium or Alumina.[28] Check a materia medica for the distinguishing features.

Homeopathy's success with infectious dis-eases made its early reputation. In the nineteenth century, the death rate for homeopathic patients in epidemics of cholera and yellow fever was half to an eighth of the death rate in standard/allopathic medicine.[29] Many infectious dis-eases today are **children's dis-eases**, some of which can be serious. For measles, Pulsatilla is the number one remedy. Also use Aconite early, and Belladonna after the rash has erupted. When the onset is gradual and the child apathetic, the remedy is Gelsemium, and Euphrasia is used when there are eye symptoms and nasal discharge. Bryonia measles have chest involvement and a dry, painful cough. For rubella or German measles, use Aconite, Belladonna, Ferrum phos or Pulsatilla. Belladonna is the first remedy for mumps, and Rhus tox for chicken pox, which can be especially serious in adults.[30] Sore throats are treated homeopathically with Belladonna, Arsenicum, Rhus tox, Mercurius, Hepar sulph, Lachesis, Apis or Phytolacca.[31] Again, consult a materia medica for the closest symptom match.

Weakness remaining after a dis-ease is sometimes treated with a homeopathically potentized remedy of that dis-ease, as Varicellinum (chicken pox), Parotidinum (mumps) or Influenzium (flu virus). The remedy gives the woman's immune system a boost and helps her shake the remaining dis-ease symptoms. Several remedies are possible, according to symptoms, for aftereffects of the flu and also for lingering respiratory symptoms. Talk to an experienced homeopath about these; it gets complicated.

Women's **menstrual** and PMS symptoms are indications for

homeopathy, as well. Magnesia phosphorica (Mag phos) and Colocynthis are used frequently for menstrual cramps if they are without other symptoms. Mag phos is indicated when cramping is relieved by warmth, and by pressure when bending forward. Colocynthis is similar, but the emphasis is on relief when curling up and pressing into the abdomen. There is anger and irritability with Colocynthis.[32] When pain is intense, try Belladonna, especially when motion worsens it. If the woman is actually doubled over with pain, Cimicfuga may be the remedy (or Colocynthis or Nux vomica are others). The pains seem to move from side to side in the abdomen, and there is pain also in the lower back.

Chamomila is the remedy for emotional aspects of PMS, irritability, criticalness, anger along with menstrual cramps that feel like labor pains. Pulsatilla in PMS is for depression, moodiness and tears but less anger. The woman may also have pain, dizziness, faintness, nausea, vomiting, diarrhea, back pain or headaches with Pulsatilla. If symptoms cease as soon as flow begins, try Lachesis, and Caulophyllum is used when there are bad premenstrual cramps that end with the flow, but end less suddenly than with Lachesis.[33]

Discomforts of **menopause** are also treatable with homeopathic remedies, though woman homeopath Sidney Spinster (who edited and advised me on this chapter) feels they are chronic rather than acute issues, requiring a trained homeopath's help. She lists Lachesis as the primary remedy picture used in menopause, indicated when health problems begin post-menopausally. Lachesis women feel worst physically and emotionally on waking. Their symptoms are often on the left side, and they may crave alcohol or have a tendency toward headaches or heart palpitations.[34]

Pulsatilla is a remedy for hot flashes, particularly those that leave the woman sleepless at night. The woman is thirstless and has rheumatism-type pains that change location and come suddenly to leave gradually. She has an aversion to fatty foods. Sepia is the remedy for the woman who resents her lack of health and holds resentment for other reasons. She feels mentally, emotionally and physically burnt out, feels cold much of the time, has backaches and a dragging sensation internally. She is always tired, emotionally irritable, and may have chronic constipation. Sepia women feel better after movement and exercise, and are relieved by sleep or eating. They may have palpitations that ease with brisk walking. Squid is a rarer remedy that benefits a woman with some of the Sepia symptoms, but she is less irritable and tired. Her work seems more difficult to her lately, and she tends to impatience and perfectionism, but is less angry than the women who benefits from

Sepia.[35]

Natrum mur is another remedy used for menopause effects. Women positive for this homeopathic remedy suffer from grief and sometimes anger or a long-term grudge. They are fiercely independent but are sensitive to criticism or ridicule from others, and are oversensitized to light. They may have low blood sugar, hypoglycemia, adrenal exhaustion, hyperthyroidism or anorexia. In menopause or otherwise (no remedy is age-specific), they suffer profuse vaginal discharges and may have severe headaches near their periods.

Other menopause remedies to consider are Calcarea carbonica or Sulphur, and less often Apis, Graphites, Phosphorus or Psorinum.[36] Remedies in menopause follow emotional states primarily, and the woman's physical symptoms respond when the remedy correct for her emotional situation is found. Read the materia medica carefully on these to pick the closest symptom fit and seek the advice of an experienced homeopath if possible.

The remedy picture for Natrum mur continues into healing **headaches and migraines**, though Belladonna is a remedy to check out first. The woman with a Natrum mur headache fits the picture above and is often in menopause, waking with the migraine and vision aberrations that lessen later in the day, but leave her feeling unwell all over. The headache is worse during menstruation, and she is highly stressed and has salt cravings. Silicea headaches start at the back of the neck and travel up the head to the right temple. Sick feelings and sweating go with it and cold winds make it worse. Using a hot water bottle gives relief.[37] The remedies that follow are more typical.

For migraines, Gelsemium or Sanguinaria headaches also begin at the back of the neck or head, and Sanguinaria headaches are right-sided. The visual disturbances of migraine and the tightness of muscle contraction headaches are Gelsemium symptoms. The woman with this headache is aggravated by light, motion, jarring and noise and wants to be left alone. Sleep or urination ease this headache, and she feels tired, heavy and apathetic with it; her eyes droop. A Sanguinaria headache is also right-sided, beginning in the back of the head and moving forward, settling on the right side or right eye. There is splitting, throbbing, knifelike pain with nausea relieved by vomiting. These headaches are cyclic migraines, and Sanguinaria is the remedy for the classic migraine pattern. Iris is also for cycle migraines affecting one side of the forehead, usually the right side, with visual aberrations and disturbances. There is nausea and vomiting, but vomiting worsens it (unlike Sanguinaria), and walking outdoors in fresh air helps.

For other types of headaches, Belladonna is used where there is throbbing, intense pain and extreme environmental sensitivity. The pain starts and ends suddenly, and motion worsens it; there may be dilated pupils and a high fever. These headaches are made better by sitting but worse by lying down or by climbing or descending stairs. Bryonia headaches are characterized by sensitivity to motion; any movement worsens it. Slight touch worsens it but heavier pressure on the pain area helps, and they are worse in the morning, usually just after getting up. The pain is a steady ache often centered in the forehead, and there may be nausea, vomiting or constipation with it.

In Nux vomica headaches (not usually migraines), the cause is often overeating, overuse of alcohol, coffee or medications, or overexhaustion. This is the morning-after headache, with sick stomach, queasiness, nausea or vomiting, and a sour taste in the mouth. Excessive mental exertion can also bring on a Nux headache, which is worse on first getting up and is aggravated by motion. Headaches responding to Pulsatilla come after meals, especially after eating fatty foods. There is indigestion, nausea and vomiting, and this headache can be menstrually related. The Pulsatilla remedy picture is for a throbbing headache, usually in the forehead or on one side, but the pain may shift. The woman is gentle and sensitive, and may weep from the pain; she wants others near her. Spigelia headaches are neurological, characterized by stiff neck and shoulders and severe pain in, behind and around the woman's eyes. The headache settles over her left eye.[38]

Homeopathy in **pregnancy** is sometimes complex, but here are a few simpler remedies as examples. Unlike prescription drugs, homeopathic remedies are safe for both pregnant woman and the unborn child.[39] A suggestion for morning sickness is for Aconite and Bryonia in 3x potency given together every half hour (classical homeopathy uses only one remedy at a time). In childbirth, Pulsatilla can turn a breech baby (if indicated), and Caulophyllum (blue cohosh, in potency only) strengthens the uterus and is used in labor to help dilation and contractions. Caulophyllum shortens labor and is likely to bring on delivery quickly. Some homeopaths recommend that it be used in the last two weeks of pregnancy routinely, while others feel it should not be given until labor starts and then only when symptoms indicate. Women who are scattered and frightened, saying "I can't do it" in labor benefit from Cimicfuga. Belladonna or Chamomila in labor is given for extreme agitation or pain.

After delivery, Arnica is used for exhaustion and afterpain, especially for muscular aches in the mother. If the labor has been difficult and with tearing of tissues, try Calendula in potency, and Arnica or Bellis Perrenis for internal injuries and torn perineum. External application of Calendula tincture (1:10 to 1:20 dilution in saline or water) speeds tissue healing—try a spray bottle of 1:10 dilution. To help a slow starting newborn breathe, Antimonium tart is used for phlegm blocking respiration, along with suction to clear the passages. Carbo veg is used for a baby who is cold and blue. If the baby is bruised or cold and stiff, homeopathic midwives use Arnica to help her overcome the birth trauma, using the remedy in liquid form with an eyedropper.[40]

In **skin and allergy** dis-eases, homeopaths believe that chemical suppression of symptoms causes greater dis-ease, as in a skin rash suppressed with cortisone that turns into asthma. In Hering's Law, a skin dis-ease is less serious than an internal one, and suppressing the rash drives the dis-ease inward, thus worsening the symptoms. This holds true also for the runny nose type of allergies, that may be driven inward by antihistamines. Self-help for allergies and rashes is limited in homeopathy, with the emphasis on constitutional remedies. For long-term remedies specific to the individual and requiring case taking and analysis consult an expert homeopath. Some suggestions for acute issues are given below.

For eczema or rashes in infants and children, try Graphites for oozing rashes, Petroleum or Sulphur for eczema on the face, neck, feet and/or hands.[41] A Graphites rash is oozing and sticky, with itching worse at night and for warmth. Sulphur is a remedy for any sort of rash, if the rest of the remedy picture fits the child or woman. Itching is worse at night when the person is warm. Homeopaths often consider eczema a food allergy. For poison ivy or poison oak rashes, use Rhus tox (potentized poison ivy) when there is pus in the vessicles, or Rhus diversiloba (potentized poison oak) when the vessicles are filled with clear fluid. Burning eruptions that itch and are worsened by scratching, open air, night or being in bed are Rhus rashes. They have inflamed, fluid-filled blisters, and the woman is anxious, restless and irritable. If the rash is blistered and inflamed but less burning, try Croton tig. These rashes are worse on the scalp, near the eyes, or on the genitals.

Anacardium rashes are large, fluid-filled blisters, often on the face. A rash that responds to Bryonia is dry, fine bumps on the skin, usually on the face, and the woman is irritable, wanting to be left alone. A dry, brownish-reddish rash with scaling, made worse by being warm in bed, though better in a warm room, responds to

Sepia. There may be small blisters here but not large ones. For all of these rashes, use diluted Calendula tincture externally to soothe and heal the skin, once the right remedy starts the rash to clear. For hives, try Apis or Urtica urens.[42]

With any of these remedy pictures, read the materia medica, choosing the remedy that closest fits your symptoms. When using the materia medica, remember that every symptom listed will not be applicable to every woman using that remedy. Pick the remedy/ remedy picture that contains all or most of a woman's symptoms, particularly the emotional ones no matter what the healing issue is.

Vaginitis and candida albicans/yeast infections are also treatable with homeopathic remedies for self-healing, but experienced homeopathic advice may be needed here. As in other homeopathic healing issues, the name of the infection is unimportant as the remedies are chosen for the symptoms. Three major remedy suggestions are Pulsatilla, Sepia and Natrum mur, used when the woman fits the personality/emotional type of the remedy.[43] Pulsatilla infection symptoms include a creamy white or yellow discharge, irritating or not. The woman may be pregnant or young, and lying down increases the discharge. Sepia is the remedy for women who have a yellowish or greenish discharge with an odor, usually worse at midcycle or just before menses. There is a bearing down sensation, and the discharge is usually more profuse in the morning. Though often a remedy for menopause, if a child has vaginitis, the remedy is probably Sepia. Vaginitis responsive to Natrum mur is profuse and watery. See the other descriptions for Sepia and Natrum mur.

Other suggestions for homeopathic remedies for vaginitis include Calcarea carbonica, which describes a thick white or yellow gushing discharge and intense itching. Graphites is the remedy for thin, burning, white discharges that come in gushes, increased in the morning and by walking. There may be back pain or abdominal tenseness. Kreosote vaginitis includes raw soreness of the genitals which become red and swollen. There is an odor that increases on standing or in the morning. The remedy is Nitric acid if the discharge is irritating and with an odor. There is greenish, brownish, flesh-colored or transparent stringy mucous, and the infection usually follows menstruation. Borax describes discharge that is clear, thick and white, like paste or egg white that may be irritating or not. A sensation of warmth accompanies the flow, which may be worse at midcycle.[44]

Homeopathy is a complex and fascinating area of women's healing, and the woman particularly drawn to detail and in-depth study is most suited to it. The process of matching a remedy to a healing need is often an involved one, using old books with archaic language to meet modern requirements. Inquisitiveness, scholarship and careful research are necessary in homeopathic healing, with patience and precision. As in other healing methods, there is still room for—and need for—women's intuition in the process. While the women's movement is only beginning to work with homeopathy, more homeopaths are needed and will come. It's a healing system worthy of women's remembering.

Says homeopathic practitioner Sidney Spinster:

> Homeopathy can help us survive patriarchy by increasing that part of our freedom which we carry around inside us. It helps us overcome unhelpful patterns of response to 'stress', oppression, pollution, etc. For example, a woman who experiences repeated grief may become walled off from other people, be unable to cry in front of others, be terrified of humiliation and get bad migraine headaches. The appropriate remedy will take that woman back to the state she was in prior to the griefs—when she had a choice whether or not she wanted to be intimate with someone and whether she wanted to 'let go' in front of others or not.

> Homeopathy can't do much to increase external freedom from oppression, pollution, radiation, etc. It will not save us from nuclear war. Individual healing must be coupled with revolution, and the healing of our wimmin's communities.

Because most women are more familiar with herb/substance names than with the latin ones, the following list defines some commonly used homeopathic remedies. The connections with herbalism become clear in this and are interesting to note.

Aconite - Monk's Hood
Agaricus - Amanita
Alumina - Aluminium
Anacardium - Marking Nut
Antimonium Tart - Tartar Emetic
Apis - Bee Venum
Aranea didema - Spider Venom
Arnica - Leopard's Bane
Arsenicum Album - Arsenious Acid
Avena Sativa - Oat
Bacillinum - Tuberculosis
Badiaga - Fresh Water Sponge
Baptisia - Wild Indigo
Belladonna - Deadly Nightshade

Bellis Perennis - Daisy
Berberis - Barberry
Borax - Borate of Sodium
Bryonia - Wild Hops
Cadmium - Cadmic Sulphate
Calcarea Carbonica - Lime Carbonate
Calendula - Marigold
Cantharis - Spanish Fly
Carbo Veg - Vegetable Charcoal
Carcinosin - Cancer
Caulophyllum - Blue Cohosh
Causticum - Tinctura acris sine Kali
Chamomila - German Chamomile
China - Quinine, Peruvian Bark
Cimicfuga - Black Snake Root
Cocculus - Indian Cockle
Colchium - Meadow Saffron
Colocynthis - Bitter Cucumber
Conium - Poison Hemlock
Croton Tiglium - Croton Oil Seed
Dulcamara - Bittersweet
Eupatorium Perfoliatum - Thoroughwort
Euphrasia - Eyebright
Ferrum Phoshoricum - Phosphate of Iron
Gelsemium - Yellow Jasmine
Graphites - Black Lead
Hepar Sulph - Calcium Sulphide
Influenzium - Flu Virus
Ipecac - Ipecac Root
Iris Versicolor - Blue Flag
Kali Bichromium - Bichromate of Potash
Kali Carbonica - Carbonate of Potassium
Kali Hydriodicum - Iodide of Potassium
Kali Muriaticum - Chloride of Potassium
Kali Sulphuricum - Potassium Sulphate
Kreosote - Beechwood Kreosote
Lachesis - Snake Venom
Lilium Tigrinum - Tiger Lily
Lycopodium - Club Moss
Magnesia Phosphorica - Phosphate of Magnesia
Mercurius - Mercury
Muriatic Acid - Muriatic Acid
Natrum Mur - Table Salt

Nitric Acid - Nitric Acid
Nux Vomica - Poison Nut
Opium - Opium Poppy
Parotidinum - Mumps
Petroleum - Crude Oil
Phosphorus - Phosphorus
Phosphoricum Acidum - Phosphoric Acid
Phytolacca - Pokeroot
Platina - Platinum
Podophyllum - May Apple
Psorinum - Scabies
Pulsatilla - Wind Flower
Rhus Diversiloba - Poison Oak
Rhus Toxicodendron - Poison Ivy
Sabina - Savine
Sanguinaria - Bloodroot
Sarsaparilla - Smilax
Secale Cornutum - Ergot
Sepia - Cuttlefish Ink
Silicea - Silica
Spigelia - Pinkroot
Spongia - Sponge
Staphysagria - Stavesacre
Sulphur - Sulphur
Syphilnum - Syphilis
Thuja - Arbor Vitae
Trifolium Pratense - Red Clover
Urtica Urens - Stinging Nettles
Varicellinum - Chicken Pox
Veratrum Album - White Hellebore

NOTES

1. Sandra Chase, MD, *Homeopathy, A Brief Overview*, (Washington, DC, National Center for Homeopathy, 1981), pamphlet, p. 1.

2. Dana Ullman, *Homeopathy: Medicine for the 21st century*, (Berkeley, CA, N. Atlantic Books, 1988), p. 7.

3. *Ibid.*, p. 33.

4. Margery Blackie, MD, *The Patient, Not the Cure: The Challenge of Homeopathy*, (Santa Barbara, CA, Woodbridge Press, 1976), pp. 13–18. This history is told in most homeopathy books.

5. Dana Ullman, *Homeopathy: Medicine for the 21st Century*, pp. 33–35.

6. Stephen Cummings, FNP and Dana Ullman, MPH, *Everybody's Guide to Homeopathic Medicines*, (Los Angeles, Jeremy Tarcher, Inc., 1984), p. 15. This information is also repeated in most homeopathy books.

7. Malcolm Hulke, *The Encyclopedia of Alternative Medicine and Self-Help*, (New York, Schocken Books, 1979), p. 118.

8. Stephen Cummings and Dana Ullman, *Everybody's Guide to Homeopathic Medicines*, pp. 18–19, and Dana Ullman, *Homeopathy: Medicine for the 21st Century*, p. 17.

9. Dana Ullman, *Homeopathy: Medicine for the 21st Century*, pp. 25–28.

10. Stephen Cummings and Dana Ullman, *Everybody's Guide to Homeopathic Medicines*, p. 25.

11. *Ibid.*

12. *Ibid.*, pp. 25–26.

13. Dana Ullman, *Homeopathy: Medicine for the 21st Century*, p. 41.

14. *Ibid.*, p. 47.

15. *Ibid.*, pp. 48–49.

16. Stephen Cummings and Dana Ullman, *Everybody's Guide to Homeopathic Medicines*, pp. 41–42.

17. Dana Ullman, *Homeopathy: Medicine for the 21st Century*, p. 133.

18. Lawrence Badgley, MD, *Healing AIDS Naturally*, (San Bruno, CA, Human Energy Press, 1987), p. 147.

19. *Ibid.*, pp. 149–151.

20. Margery Blackie, *The Patient, Not the Cure*, pp. 53–56.

21. Stephen Cummings and Dana Ullman, *Everybody's Guide to Homeopathic Medicines*, pp. 71–83.

22. *Ibid.*, pp. 60–65.

23. Dana Ullman, *Homeopathy: Medicine for the 21st Century*, p. 130.

24. Margery Blackie, *The Patient, Not the Cure*, p. 180.

25. Dana Ullman, *Homeopathy: Medicine for the 21st Century*, pp. 110–111.

26. Stephen Cummings and Dana Ullman, *Everybody's Guide to Homeopathic Medicines*, pp. 155–158.

27. *Ibid.*, pp. 131–137, and 142.

28. Margerie Blackie, *The Patient, Not the Cure*, p. 99.

29. Dana Ullman, *Homeopathy: Medicine for the 21st Century*, p. 126.

30. Stephen Cummings and Dana Ullman, *Everybody's Guide to Homeopathic Medicines*, pp. 96–105.

31. Dana Ullman, *Homeopathy: Medicine for the 21st Century*, p. 127.

32. *Ibid.*, p. 110.

33. Stephen Cummings and Dana Ullman, *Everybody's Guide to Homeopathic Medicines*, pp. 151–154.

34. Dana Ullman, *Homeopathy: Medicine for the 21st Century*, pp. 117–118.

35. Margery Blackie, *The Patient, Not the Cure*, pp. 121–124.

36. Dana Ullman, *Homeopathy: Medicine for the 21st Century*, pp. 117–118.

37. Margery Blackie, *The Patient, Not the Cure*, p. 113.

38. Stephen Cummings and Dana Ullman, *Everybody's Guide to Homeopathic Medicines*, pp. 172–177.

39. Dana Ullman, *Homeopathy: Medicine for the 21st Century*, p. 78.

40. *Ibid.*, pp. 80–86.

41. Margery Blackie, *The Patient, Not the Cure*, pp. 106–107.

42. Stephen Cummings and Dana Ullman, *Everybody's Guide to Homeopathic Medicines*, pp. 180–181.

43. Dana Ullman, *Homeopathy: Medicine for the 21st Century*, pp. 112–115.

44. Stephen Cummings and Dana Ullman, *Everybody's Guide to Homeopathic Medicines*, pp. 148–149.

Chapter Ten

———————◯———————

Flower Remedies and Gem Elixirs

Flower and gemstone elixirs are similar to homeopathic remedies but are not the same in preparation or intent. They heal directly, not by the law of similars, and they heal emotional dis-eases from the unseen aura levels. In flower remedies or gem elixirs, the blossom or gemstone is placed in distilled or spring water and exposed to sunlight or moonlight to potentize it. This creates a mother tincture that is diluted or may remain undiluted with either gemstones or flowers. The flowers or stones heal by their essence or vibrations entering the liquid that holds them, and the essence transfers to the woman's aura when she takes the remedy. The four elements and spirit that compose the plant or gem enter the remedies or elixirs. A plant grows in earth and air, is watered by rain and nurtured by the sun and moon, and the same four elements go into the formation of gemstones and crystals by fire in the earth. Potentized by gentle natural means, usually without the succussion used in homeopathy, these remedies are important women's healing tools. Gaining popularity in the last several years, flower remedies and gemstone elixirs have earned wide use.

Flower remedies were currently discovered by Edward Bach (1886–1936), an English homeopath and physician, but their use has pre-historic matriarchal beginnings. The potentizing of elixirs was an early healing secret, originating before recorded history. The healing wells of England and Europe were potentized by putting specific leaves or nuts into them before drinking the waters.[1] The ancient healing wells were places of Persephone, the maiden Goddess of the witch-healers, and they still exist, though most are covered and unknown today. In the 1930s Bach discovered that certain wildflower blossoms, picked and prepared only in full bloom and on clear sunny days could be potentized to heal emotional dis-eases. His specific method of potentization is not described, except that they are prepared in water and sunlight. No toxic plants or herbs are used, none that produce any sort of side effects. Most were chosen psychically, as Bach was allegedly so sensitive he could determine a flower's use simply by putting it in his mouth.[2]

Thirty-eight remedies in all were discovered and chosen, and given careful research. They heal mental and emotional dis-ease states, which Bach (and women's healing) define as the basic cause of all dis-ease. In this era of high speed and high stress, they have found an important place in women's healing as a rediscovered remnant of ancient women's methods: the healing of negative emotions can heal physical dis-ease.

Earlier in this book is a discussion of emotional sources of dis-ease and the work done by Louise Hay with releasing negative emotions for physical healing. She works at an emotional and mental body level. Flower remedies also work on the nonphysical levels of dis-ease and healing, specifically on the emotional, mental and spiritual bodies. A woman would take a flower essence for fear, using the remedy to help her release fear and its effects from her aura. She would not take the remedy for a skin issue or stomach ulcer caused by the fear, but releasing the fear will heal her skin and ulcer. As in homeopathy, it is the essence of the plant matter, its nonphysical vibration, that is the agent for healing women's nonphysical Being.

Flower remedies and gemstone elixirs work on the level of women's Goddess-within to clear imbalances and disharmonies. Since vibration/energy travels from the spiritual level through the mental and emotional to the etheric double, from which the physical level is influenced, clearing disharmonies in the outer levels clears them in the physical body. Negative emotions lodged in the emotional body or negative thought patterns stuck in the mental body prevent Goddess-within from manifesting clearly in women. The result is dis-ease, which begins in the unseen levels, then manifests on the seen one. Flower remedies and gem elixirs work to change the negative vibration, open the blocks and establish aura balance and healing harmony. They heal dis-ease or prevent its manifesting. Similar to homeopathic remedies, flower remedies are made from plants chosen specifically for their pure and positive energies and aura influence.

Flower remedies are purchased at healthfood or herb stores. They cost about ten dollars for a tiny vial of the concentrated essence preserved in alcohol. The small amount goes a long way, however, as only two drops are used (four of Rescue Remedy) placed under the tongue or in a glass of spring water, herb tea or fruit juice, (but not in coffee, pop or alcoholic beverages). No restrictions are placed on using them with other substances, as in the items that can antidote a homeopathic remedy, but in my experience coffee will antidote them, and possibly peppermint or camphor, when used too closely together. Use the remedies first thing in the morning, last thing at night and twice in between, usually midway between meals. Avoid taking them within twenty to thirty minutes of eating (this is also true of homeopathic remedies). They can be taken more often in acute issues, as often as every few minutes if needed. Some women may be interested in developing home potentizing, thereby saving the cost, as these are common flowers. The process is described under gem elixirs.

Another way of making up the remedies is to prepare them in a brown eyedropper bottle in a dilution with alcohol or cider vinegar and spring water. The recipe for this is to use a one-ounce bottle, filling it three quarters of the way with spring water (not distilled water), and adding two drops each of the chosen remedy or remedies. The bottle is then filled to the top with about a teaspoonful of brandy or cider vinegar. (The vinegar leaves a sour taste that takes getting used to.) Little alcohol is involved, as the mixture is used in drops, but the alcohol or vinegar is a preservative. When a stock bottle, as it's called, is used, the dose is four drops four times daily, usually taken under the tongue.[3] Keep the eyedropper from touching the tongue, or rinse it afterwards, to prevent saliva from contaminating the remedy. Some sources list five and others list nine for the top number of remedies that can be used in one stock bottle, but one remedy works well too and is recommended. Unlike homeopathy that uses one remedy at a time, more flower remedies may be used in one dilution. I have had better success with full doses than with using the stock bottle method, but other women prefer the stock bottles. The remedies are used for at least a month and then evaluated.

Flower essences work with emotional issues, rather than physical dis-eases, and are the only method of women's healing designed specifically for this. When the remedies are taken in need, the result is a sigh of relief, particularly when using Rescue Remedy in a crisis. When the remedy is unneeded or the wrong one, it has no effect. It is totally nontoxic—nothing happens. Each remedy picture for a flower essence establishes an emotional state or thought pattern. Women pick one or more that fit their individual needs. Establishment medicine ignores flower essences, but a few MDs use them and attempt to describe their actions in psychodynamic terms which seem somewhat silly. The fact is that neither Bach nor anyone else knows why or how these essences work, but only that they do work. Healers using the aura theory are probably closest to the truth. Women who find their emotional or mental discomfort or dis-ease described by a flower remedy description find relief in using the remedy. Chronic issues change gradually, when using the stock bottle method for a period of time, a month to six weeks or longer. The change is natural, gentle and almost imperceptible. Acute crisis issues ease in a matter of minutes.

Unlike homeopathic remedy pictures, flower remedy pictures are clear-cut and very simple. There are only thirty-eight, as compared to thousands of homeopathic choices, and the descriptions are focused totally on emotional healing. To find the right remedy, read over all the descriptions, then pick the one(s) that reflect your own feelings, issues or thought patterns that you choose to change. Choosing to change a negative pattern is half the healing. Make up a stock bottle containing the correct remedy and use it four times a day for at least a month to six weeks to start. Designing affirmations to use with the remedies is also positive. At the end of the time, go back to the remedy description and compare it with your present emotional situation. If more time is needed, continue the remedy. If the pattern has changed, either continue a while longer, seek another remedy that applies, or stop completely. If the new emotional pattern is not sustained, start the remedy again.

If a remedy doesn't work, there are several possible reasons. One is you may not have been taking it long enough. Or the remedy may be working but with such gentle changes that the woman's awareness hasn't come yet. Another reason for seeming failure may be karmic—that it's not time to heal a particular issue or it isn't meant to be healed in this lifetime. In karmic theory, dis-eases are considered learning situations, but the learning may also be in taking the initiative to heal it. Take into account, too, the state of a patriarchal world that oppresses women, non-whites, the disabled, gays and the poor so heavily, and pollutes so heavily, that any healing is that much harder. Failure can also happen when the woman, consciously or not, chooses to keep her symptoms or disease; she may be getting something she needs from doing so. Occasionally a woman is so sure that a remedy is useless that she blocks its potential for healing.[4] Consider these possibilities, meditate on them and ask your Goddess-within what to do next.

The thirty-eight flower remedies are divided into seven categories, of four to eight remedies in each. The categories are remedies

Bach Flower Remedies

Agrimony For those not wishing to burden others with their troubles and who cover up their suffering behind a cheerful facade. They are distressed by argument or quarrel, and may seek escape from pain and worry through the use of drugs and alcohol.

Aspen For those who experience vague fears and anxieties of unknown origin, they are often apprehensive.

Beech For those who while desiring perfection easily find fault with people and things. Critical and at times intolerant, they may overreact to small annoyances or idiosyncracies of others.

Centaury For those who are over-anxious to please, often weak willed and easily exploited or dominated by others. As a result they may neglect their own particular interests.

Cerato For those who lack confidence in their own judgment and decisions. They constantly seek the advice of others and may often be misguided.

Cherry Plum For fear of losing mental and physical control, of doing something desperate. May have impulses to do things thought or known to be wrong.

Chestnut Bud For those who fail to learn from experience, repeating the same patterns or mistakes again and again.

Chicory For those who are overfull of care for others and need to direct and control those close to them. Always finding something to correct or put right.

Clematis For those who tend to live in the future, lack concentration, are daydreamers, drowsy or spacey and have a half-hearted interest in their present circumstances.

Crab Apple For those who may feel something is not quite clean about themselves, or have a fear of being contaminated. For feelings of shame or poor self image. For example, thinking oneself not attractive for one reason or another. When necessary, may be taken to assist in detoxification, for example, during a cold or while fasting.

Elm For those who at times may experience momentary feelings of inadequacy, being overwhelmed by their responsibilities.

Gentian For those who become easily discouraged by small delays or hindrances. This may cause self-doubt.

Gorse For feelings of hopelessness and futility. When there is little hope of relief.

Heather For those who seek the companionship of anyone who will listen to their troubles. They are generally not good listeners and have difficulty being alone for any length of time.

Holly To be used when troubled by negative feelings such as envy, jealousy, suspicion, revenge. Vexations of the heart, states indicating a need for more love.

Honeysuckle For those dwelling in the past, nostalgia, homesickness, always talking about the good old days, when things were better.

Hornbeam For the Monday morning feeling of not being able to face the day. For those feeling some part of the body or mind needs strengthening. Constant fatigue, tiredness.

Impatiens For those quick in tought and action, who require all things to be done without delay. They are impatient with people who are slow and often prefer to work alone.

Larch For those who, despite being capable, lack self confidence or feel inferior. Anticipating failure, they often refuse to make a real effort to succeed.

Mimulus For fear of known things, such as heights, water, the dark, other people, of being alone, etc.

Mustard For deep gloom which comes on for no known reason, sudden melancholia or heavy sadness. Will lift just as suddenly.

At A Glance Reference

Oak For those who struggle on despite despondency from hardships, even when ill and overworked, they never give up.

Olive For mental and physical exhaustion, sapped vitality with no reserve. This may come on after an illness or personal ordeal.

Pine For those who feel they should do or should have done better, who are self-reproachful or blame themselves for the mistakes of others. Hardworking people who suffer much from the faults they attach to themselves, they are never satisfied with their success.

Red Chestnut For those who find it difficult not to be overly concerned or anxious for others, always fearing something wrong may happen to those they care for.

Rock Rose For those who experience states of terror, panic and hysteria; also when troubled by nightmares.

Rock Water For those who are very strict with themselves in their daily living. They are hard masters to themselves struggling toward some ideal or to set an example for others. This would include strict adherence to a living style or to religious, personal or social disciplines.

Scleranthus For those unable to decide between two things, first one seeming right then the other. Often presenting extreme variations in energy or mood swings.

Star of Bethlehem For grief, trauma, loss. For the mental and emotional effect during and after a trauma.

Sweet Chestnut For those who feel they have reached the limits of their endurance. For those moments of deep despair when the anguish seems to be unbearable.

Vervain For those who have strong opinions and who usually need to have the last word, always teaching or philosophizing. When taken to an extreme they can be argumentative and overbearing.

Vine For those who are strong willed. Leaders in their own right who are unquestionably in charge. However, when taken to an extreme they may become dictatorial.

Walnut Assists in stabilizing emotional upsets during transition periods, such as puberty, adolescence, menopause. Also helps to break past links and emotionally adjust to new beginnings such as moving, changing or taking a new job, beginning or ending a relationship.

Water Violet For those who are gentle, independent, aloof and self-reliant, who do not interfere in the affairs of others, and when ill or in trouble prefer to bear their difficulties alone.

White Chestnut For constant and persistent unwanted thoughts, such as mental arguments, worries or repetitious thoughts that prevent peace-of-mind, and disrupt concentration.

Wild Oat For the dissatisfaction with not having succeeded in one's career or life goal. When there is unfulfilled ambition, career uncertainty or boredom with one's present position or station in life.

Wild Rose For those, who for no apparent reason, have resigned themselves to their circumstances. Having become indifferent, little effort is made to improve things or find joy.

Willow For those who have suffered some circumstance or misfortune, which they feel was unfair or unjust. As a result they become resentful and bitter toward life or toward those who they feel were at fault.

NOTE: Conditions requiring proper medical attention should be referred to a physician.

Bach Centre USA, *The Bach Flower Remedies* (Windemere, NY, Bach Centre USA, 1983), pp. 8–9.

for fear, uncertainty, insufficient interest in present circumstances, loneliness, over-sensitivity to influences and ideas, despondency or despair, and over-care for the welfare of others.[5] Within the categories, most women find a remedy or remedies that are helpful to their issues and needs. Loneliness, despair, grief, burnout, or lack of self-confidence are emotions common to everyone at sometime or another. When an emotion of this sort is not temporary, and becomes an obstacle to well-being, the time has come to change it. Likewise, in crisis situations, when the feelings are acute and painful, the remedies will bring relief and make the pain more transient.

The first category is for fear, and the remedy choices are Rock Rose, Mimulus, Cherry Plum, Aspen and Red Chestnut. **Rock Rose** is used for emergencies, often combined with other remedies as in Rescue Remedy. Terror, panic, hysteria or nightmares are indications for this remedy, as are accidents or sudden illness. If the woman is unconscious, place a few drops on her lips; if a child awakens with night terrors, give her two drops in a glass of water. The remedy is for any sort of fear at gut level, and any sort of panic.

Mimulus is also for fear, but of a different sort. This is a fear of known things in everyday life, secret and unspoken dreads. There are anxieties of the dark, of dying, of cancer, of driving or car accidents, of poverty or being alone. The Mimulus woman is frightened and burdened by her fears to the point where life is not enjoyable. A sensitive, artistic woman who feels things deeply, she may feel shy around others, experiencing stress headaches or stage fright. She seldom talks about her fears unless asked.

Aspen fears are similar to Mimulus, with the difference that the Mimulus woman knows what she is afraid of and the Aspen woman does not. In Aspen, there are undefined anxieties, haunting and inexplicable, yet terrifying.

Cherry Plum is another remedy for fear, different again from the fears of Rock Rose, Mimulus or Aspen. The remedy picture for Cherry Plum is the woman who fears she will do some wrong, who sees the image of wrong-doing and it horrifies her, yet she fears she will do it. She fears a nervous breakdown and her self-control is at the breaking point; she may feel suicidal. The woman fears her own subconscious processes and holds it all inside, and her anxiety may come from suppressing her spiritual or psychic growth.

In **Red Chestnut** fears, the remedy picture is of a woman who is anxious for others, not herself, fearing terrible things will happen to someone she loves. She is a strong empath/telepath, and transmits her caring and anxieties. Her fears can draw negativities to those she fears for, or create a dependent relationship that is not positive. The mother who lives through her child is an example. Remember in the case of all fears, that what you think you draw to you, and negative thought-forms can manifest fears on the physical plane. The use of the flower remedy that describes a woman's fear helps her to release it, changing negative thought-forms to positive ones.

Uncertainty is the second category of flower remedy pictures, with Cerato, Scleranthus, Gentian, Gorse, Hornbeam and Wild Oat as the remedies. **Cerato** strengthens a woman's inner voice/Goddess-within, and is for the woman who is unable to accept intellectually what she knows intuitively. A Cerato woman is afraid to make her own decisions, and asks others' help and advice constantly. The remedy helps her to accept what she knows inside, and to depend on herself instead of on others.

Scleranthis is the remedy for a woman who can't decide between two choices but changes back and forth between them. She moves to extremes in emotions, moods and opinions. Not dependent on others to decide for her, as the Cerato woman is, she still can't decide or stay balanced. Her physical symptoms may also shift. The woman vascillates between extremes, physically, mentally, emotionally or spiritually. The remedy is also used in pregnancy for morning sickness.

Gentian is for the woman who is easily discouraged and who loses faith at the smallest setback. Spiritually, she would like to believe but cannot and therefore can't trust the flow and positivity of life. She is a worrier, skeptic and eternal pessimist. Depression from a known cause is also helped by Gentian, as in grief, job loss or hospitalization. Gentian women are given to intellectualizing.

Gorse is the remedy picture for a woman who has given up and believes that nothing will help her. She may have a chronic disease, chronic poverty, or simply a negative emotional state, but if she feels that nothing can help her, nothing will. With optimism, self-determination and an awareness of the learnings of karma, the woman regains her balance.

Hornbeam is the remedy for a woman who feels that life's burdens are more than she can bear or meet. She believes she needs strengthening in some part of her body, emotions, mind or spirit to be able to continue her life. Hornbeam is also for the Monday morning blues, the feeling of not being able to face the week, of being too tired to do it. Mental overexertion or boredom causes her emotional picture. She wakes up more tired than when she went to bed. The woman who works as a secretary in an office is a typical candidate for Hornbeam.

Wild Oat uncertainty differs from the other remedies for uncertainty. The woman who benefits from this remedy lacks focus and is frustrated at her unfulfilled goals, though her talents and potentials are many and varied. She starts things but loses interest though she is highly successful. She wants to do something special but she doesn't know what it is. With so many choices all of which are positive, she doesn't know what she wants. She looks without instead of within for answers.

The third category of remedy pictures is of women who have insufficient interest in their present circumstances and do not live in the here and now. The remedies include Clematis, Honeysuckle, Wild Rose, Olive, White Chestnut, Mustard and Chestnut Bud. The woman who benefits from **Clematis** is a quiet, spacey woman who lives in the future. She has hopes of better things to come, though is not fully happy now. In illness she may not work to get well or may hope passively for death. She has a hard time staying in her body, spaces out, astral projects, is absentminded or may faint. She is often a creative woman trapped in a just-for-money job.

Honeysuckle pictures a woman who lives in the past. She is stuck in the loss of a loved one or a positive life period that is gone, and regrets a decision that changed her life at that time. She is homesick, nostalgic and regretful, without hope that the present or future is as good.

A woman who is helped by **Wild Rose** is indifferent, accepting life as it is without trying to improve it. She has an underlying deep sadness and resignation, along with tiredness and chronic boredom. There seems to be no reason for her attitude.

In **Olive**, the remedy picture is of a woman who has suffered so much mentally or physically that she is too exhausted to make further efforts. A long illness or emotional ordeal can trigger this. The woman needs a lot of sleep, and any activity is an effort.

White Chestnut is the remedy to use for continuous unwanted thoughts that run round and round through the mind. The woman is a chronic worrier, maybe an insomniac, with constant mental chatter that leaves her no peace. Her mental treadmill interferes with her ability to concentrate. Meditation helps this woman, and White Chestnut is her flower remedy.

Mustard has a remedy picture of a woman who experiences times of deep depression, seemingly for no reason. The depressions come and go suddenly, and the woman's Being is in deep mourning during them. She is caught up in these moods, unable to break them and unable to hide them from others. She can see no connection between her depressions and the conditions of her life.

Chestnut Bud is the remedy for a woman who takes a long time to learn life's lessons. She repeats her mistakes over and over, without learning to avoid them. The woman is self-willed and seems selfish, with an inability to change her ideas or thought patterns. She refuses to face the issues and break her negative patterns, but Chestnut Bud and affirmations help.

There are three flower essences for loneliness—Water Violet, Impatiens and Heather. A woman positive for **Water Violet** lives quietly and generally likes being alone. She is independent, aloof, nonreceptive and unwilling to reach out to others. Rarely crying and very reserved, she appears supercilious or stuck-up to others, but in fact is not and feels isolated, separated and uninvolved. At times she withdraws.

Impatiens is for the woman who is quick-thinking and quick-acting, and expects others to be the same. She prefers to work alone, as others are too slow for her. An Impatiens woman is extroverted, makes nervous gestures, moves quickly and rapidly, is sometimes accident prone, and gets tired easily from all her anxious energy. Working well alone, she has difficulty working with others or being patient with them.

Heather loneliness is different from Impatiens or Water Violet. The Heather remedy picture is of a woman who often or constantly needs to tell someone else her problems. She is selfish and not a good listener, insisting that others listen to her. She is a compulsive talker, primarily about herself. The Heather woman is a needy child not yet able to grow up and be giving. She worries too much and makes mountains out of molehills, but her distress is real. Women who are unconscious energy sappers are the Heather type.

The fifth category of flower remedies is for those women who are oversensitive to others' influence or ideas. Agrimony, Centaury, Walnut and Holly are included in it. An **Agrimony** remedy picture is of a woman who conceals inner torment behind her appearance of easy-going cheerfulness. She does anything possible to avoid confrontations and to keep the peace, denies or minimizes her problems, and looks for activities and good times to distract her from her issues. This is the woman who may turn to alcohol or drugs to cope; she is unable to ask for help or admit difficulties, and going it alone is unbearable. She holds a pattern of inner pain and loneliness from childhood.

Centaury is the remedy for a woman who is over-anxious to serve. She is a giver who submerges her Being in others' needs willingly, while denying her own needs and growth. Overworked and overtired, she is a passive woman who has not yet learned to assert herself, a gentle and sensitive woman with a sense of service and duty that is overdone. Often she is a woman just opening spiritually or psychically who has not yet found her balance. She may be looking for a guru, instead of looking to Goddess-within. Centaury helps her find balance and a knowledge of when to refuse.

Walnut is for a woman going through major life changes or transition periods, as at the beginnings and endings of relationships, at menarche or menopause, pregnancy, terminal illness, or on moving to a new home. The Walnut woman is easily influenced because her life is temporarily unstable and she is highly sensitive. She knows what she wants and where she's going but is temporarily led off track. She has difficulty escaping from someone else's dominant nature, or new choices are making her rethink her life. Walnut eases the transition and helps her to be clear and steady.

The **Holly** remedy picture is of a woman who is highly jealous, frustrated and discontent. She forgets that no one owns another, and that there is abundance of riches for everyone. She fears being deceived and distrusts others, and has periods of anger and rage that sometimes have physical symptoms. Supersensitive, she feels slighted and hurt. Her heart is not open, and she sees only the negative side of others, therefore drawing that to her. Holly helps open the heart chakra, and is also useful for women in terminal illnesses. The issue with Holly women is a need for more love.

There are eight flower remedies for despondency and despair: Larch, Pine, Elm, Sweet Chestnut, Star of Bethlehem, Willow, Oak and Crab Apple, and again the remedy pictures are different for each. The woman who is positive for **Larch** feels inferior to other women. She doesn't try hard enough because she feels she is not good enough; she expects failure, and the expectation creates it. The situation can be temporary or chronic and is basically a lack of self-confidence. The woman says, "I can't," but she really can. The remedy is a good one for stage fright.

In **Pine**, the issue is guilt and self-blame, something changed in women's spirituality and healing to blameless responsibility. The woman sets high standards and feels guilty if she can't live up to them; if she succeeds, she feels she could have done more, and she devalues her achievements. Her attitude is that she doesn't deserve love or other good things in life. Her system of morality may be a rigid one.

The **Elm** remedy picture is of a woman who feels overwhelmed by responsibility and temporarily inadequate to it. She has reached a point of burnout and exhaustion where there is too much work and she cannot separate herself from it. Elm helps her to go on.

Sweet Chestnut is the remedy for when things become unbearable and intolerable, and the anguish is too much to overcome. The woman is at the bottom of despair; she is not suicidal as in Cherry Plum, but her world is in chaos and there is nowhere to go. Ends are new beginnings, and Sweet Chestnut helps to turn the wheel.

Star of Bethlehem is for the numb period following great trauma that is physical, emotional, mental or spiritual. Used in Rescue Remedy, it helps release trauma from the aura to begin the healing process. The woman is dazed and in shock, a temporary but serious situation. Not seeing, not speaking or not hearing caused by emotional paralysis are helped with Star of Bethlehem, as are birth trauma in newborns, and women emerging from car accidents. It comforts and soothes pain, fright and grief.

Willow is for the woman who is bitter over the disappointments of her life. She feels unfairly treated and holds resentments, often blaming others for her misfortunes and pain. She is negative and makes demands but is not willing to give. She takes help from others without returning it. Begrudging others' good fortune, the Willow woman withdraws from activities she enjoys and is moody, touchy, spiteful or angry. She refuses to admit her negativity and refuses to change. The willow has always been Hecate's tree, and Willow helps to bring about her balance.

An **Oak** woman continues against all odds, despite despondency and hardships. She overworks and then is exhausted, but has persistence, endurance and patience. Whatever else, she goes on, not allowing her weakness from exhaustion or dis-ease to be known to others or to interfere. Her despair may be physical, emotional or mental, but she fights illness and refuses to give up.

Crab Apple is the remedy of purification and is used to help detoxify in fasts or illness. The woman is a perfectionist, magnifying any flaw and not able to see the forest for the trees. She feels unclean or impure from low self-image, feels herself contaminated by the latest flu epidemic or bacteria in a restaurant. The remedy removes negative impressions or thought forms from women who seem to attract them. It purifies, clears and decontaminates the vibrations and aura.

Over-care for the welfare of others is the last category of the seven remedy categories. It includes Chicory, Vervain, Vine, Beech and Rock Water. **Chicory** is for the woman who overcares for and overcontrols her children and loved ones. She fusses and finds things to fix, is overpossessive, and wants her people close. The remedy is also positive for the child who insists on being the center of attention, throwing tantrums and crying when she isn't noticed. The Chicory child or woman feels empty and unfulfilled, taking her fulfillment through others, manifesting it negatively as manipulation, willfulness or power-over in the name of love and caring. Her love is conditional with martyred behavior and illnesses to gain attention.

Vervain's remedy picture is overeager and fanatic, drawing others in with her enthusiasms. The woman has strong opinions and wants to have the last word, teaching others and always being right. She fights for a just cause, with a great sense of mission and a need to convert. She is anxious, swift speaking and swift moving, continuing even when exhausted or burnt out.

The **Vine** woman is capable and confident, a strong-willed leader who tends to be dictatorial. She demands obedience of women who work with her and is greedy for power, but she misuses power. Unbalanced on power-over/power-within issues, she may fawn on authorities, while dominating those she works with. In children or adults, the Vine remedy picture is of a bully, a woman who needs greater awareness.

Beech is the remedy picture for a perfectionist, intolerant of others and hard or narrowminded. The woman judges others, is unable to show understanding or empathy, and sees only what is wrong. Tense, rigid, hypercritical and often isolated from others, the woman helped by Beech may overreact to others' quirks.

In **Rock Water**, the remedy picture is of a woman who works very hard to be an example to others, a perfectionist who is hard on herself (rather than Beech who is hard on others). The woman believes that spirituality has only one road and she insists on denying portions of her inner Being (her sexuality or physical needs perhaps) in spirituality's name. Her life is highly stressed and she may be anorexic or have difficult menstruations; she lives with a variety of compulsive behaviors. Rock Water is the only flower remedy that is not a blossom, but is water from the holy wells of England, places of Persephone, the maiden Goddess. Using it changes the negative state to a positive one of balanced spirituality, high ideals, joy, inner peace, and projects brought to fulfillment. The remedy is for the crown chakra, opening it to Goddess and Goddess-within.

The last of the flower remedies is the most popular, and is called **Rescue Remedy**. It is composed of five remedies, Star of Bethlehem, Rock Rose, Impatiens, Cherry Plum and Clematis. The properties are Rock Rose for terror and panic, Star of Bethlehem for

Flower Remedy Categories

Fear

Rock Rose for terror
Mimulus for fear of known things
Aspen for fear of the unknown
Cherry Plum for fear of doing wrong
Red Chestnut fears for others

Uncertainty

Cerato for making own decisions
Scleranthis for deciding between two things
Gentian for easy discouragement and
    depression from a known cause
Gorse for a woman who has given up
Hornbeam for strengthening
Wild Oat for too many choices and lack of
    focus

Insufficient interest in the present

Clematis for living in the future
Honeysuckle for living in the past
Wild Rose for indifference
Olive for being too exhausted to care
White Chestnut for unwanted thoughts
Mustard for times of deep depression
Chestnut Bud to break negative patterns

Over sensitivity to others' influence

Agrimony for inner torment/outer cheer
Centaury for over-serving
Walnut for major life changes
Holly for jealousy

Despondency and despair

Larch for feeling inferior
Pine for guilt
Elm for burn-out
Sweet Chestnut for when things become
    intolerable
Star of Bethlehem for shock
Willow for resentment and disappointment
Crab Apple for purification

Over-care for the welfare of others

Chicory for possessiveness
Vervain for fanaticism
Vine for power-over
Beech for perfectionism over others
Rock Water for perfectionism over self

Loneliness

Water Violet for withdrawal
Impatiens for impatience
Heather for needy talking

Rescue Remedy
Five Remedies Together
for First Aid and Stress
Rock Rose for terror and panic
Star of Bethlehem for shock, trauma and
    numbness
Impatiens for tension and irritability
Cherry Plum for fear of losing control
Clematis to prevent leaving the body

shock, trauma and numbness, Impatiens for tension and irritability, Cherry Plum for fear of losing control, and Clematis to prevent passing out and keep the woman in her body.[6] Rescue Remedy comes in a bottle of concentrated liquid, as the other remedies do, or in a cream for external use. Not only for accidents and first aid, Rescue Remedy is positive for any emotional or physical trauma, stress or grief. Use it to calm down after a bad day at work, an argument or bad news, in an emergency room (for the patient and her family), and to help women working under high stress. The remedy can be used in the concentrate or made up into the stock bottle, using four drops to an ounce of spring water and alcohol preservative. Use it as often as needed, every few minutes in extreme stress, either full strength or four drops placed in a glass of water or juice.

Rescue Remedy is safe for children, pets and houseplants, as are the other remedies. For pets, place the drops in the dog or cat's water or into its mouth, and for plants use ten drops from the stock bottle in a gallon of water and water them as usual. Ten drops per gallon is the amount to also use for large animals, the drops placed in their drinking water. For infants or a woman who is unconscious, drop the remedy on her lips, gums, temples, crown, back of neck, wrists or behind her ears.[7]

Flower remedies are positive for women's healing, for the release and balancing of negative emotions. Though developed by a man in this century, the knowledge is ancient and the remedies may be a women's reclaiming. Flower essences were connected with the holy wells, Goddess healing places, giving indication of a remembering long lost. The remedies are highly effective and positive for helping women deal with the stresses of a patriarchal world. They are the only system designed specifically for emotional balance and healing.

Gemstone elixirs are very similar to flower remedies, as well as to homeopathic ones. They use gemstones, rather than flower blossoms, and are potentized to transmit the properties of the stone they are made from without destroying the gemstone. Women make them readily at home, choosing the gemstone properties they need for their physical, mental, emotional or spiritual healing issues. Working by vibration, as do flower remedies and homeopathics, gemstone essences operate on the level of the four bodies to clear women's auras and chakras of dis-ease. Since use of gemstones goes back to the matriarchies worldwide, and since there is good evidence that essences and elixirs are an ancient healing knowledge, it seems likely that gemstone essences are a women's method of healing. The skill of gem elixirs is one of the bodies of channeled knowledge being received from Atlantis and Lemuria, going back to those advanced technological civilizations that are gone.

Women who work with crystals and gemstones are aware of their positive powers of healing. They effect women's unseen aura/ energy bodies to open blocks and release dis-ease from the physical level. Stones work through the chakra system and are chosen by their colors on the principle of the doctrine of signatures. This theory states that what a stone looks like or resembles gives a clue to what it is used for. A red stone by this concept is used for healing the red root center chakra, and in the 'like cures like' theory also heals such things as fevers and blood dis-eases. (Some women choose to use opposite/complementary colors for fever—green or blue to cool it instead.) In this concept also, hematite that runs red when cut is used to stop bleeding, and since it is both black and red for the inside and outside of the womb, it is used to prevent hemorrhaging in childbirth. A stone that is yellow, the color of the sun, stimulates energy and warmth, and a stone that's green heals the heart and draws money.

Gemstones for the chakras are given in chapter one of this book, and are also discussed thoroughly in *The Women's Book of Healing*. Any good book on gemstones gives information on what stones to use for what dis-ease, and this section is primarily on using them as essences. To determine a stone's use, first look at its color, as the color of the stone matches the chakra color it works best with. After choosing the color, look for definitions and healing uses of the individual stones. Once the stone is chosen and a piece of it is available, make it into a gem elixir by the process below. What a stone does in healing is what it does in a gemstone elixir, and the process of potentizing the elixir amplifies the gemstone properties. The stone is not destroyed in the making or potentizing of the gemstone essence and it may be used repeatedly.

From Gurudas, *Gem Elixirs and Vibrational Healing*, Vol. I, (Boulder, CO, Cassandra Press, 1985),[8] the following materials are needed to make a gemstone elixir: a glass bowl, glass funnel, distilled water, glass eyedropper bottles, labels for the bottles, and the gemstone. The bowl should be clear and without designs or patterns, as patterns enter the elixir's energy. The bowl holds about twelve ounces of liquid. The funnel and eyedropper bottles, including the eyedroppers themselves are of glass also, as plastic (a petroleum product) is a contaminant to the essence. These items (new ones) are sterilized in hot water in an enameled, glass, or stainless steel pot (never aluminum) for ten minutes before using. Only distilled water is used in making essences, as the minerals in spring water would enter the elixir, and the chemicals in tap water are toxic. Both effect gem essences negatively. This is different from flower remedies that require spring water.

A small piece of gemstone is used, rather than a larger piece, and the gemstone must be rough, uncut and unpolished. Use a stone of the highest quality possible and without inclusions of other minerals. The stone that retains its matrix-base (still in the rough rock it grows in) is positive. The elixir is enhanced if the stone comes from a place known for its quality gemstones of that type, as moonstones from India or chrysocolla from Peru. Before starting, clear the stone in dry sea salt or use another form of gemstone cleansing process. Some stones are amplified by putting them in sunlight or under the full moon for a period of time before using them. Stones for the moon are moonstone, pearl, clear quartz, and other clear, opaque, white, indigo or violet gemstones. Other stones prefer sunlight, including diamonds, emeralds, fire agates, lode-stone, malachite, peridot, ruby, sapphire and the tourmalines. Stones for the 'hotter' colors respond to solar energies; stones for the 'cooler' ones to lunar. Avoid sun and use moonlight instead for amethyst or rose quartz, as they fade.

Take the cleared and sun- or moon-enhanced gemstone and place it in the bottom center of the sterilized glass bowl. A ring of clear quartz crystals outside the bowl helps to potentize the elixir. Make sure any salt is rinsed from the stone before placing it. Fill the remainder of the bowl with distilled water. Set the bowl containing the gemstone and water in the sun for about two hours, setting it on the earth rather than on concrete. Sunny days in spring are considered optimal, with a cloudless sky. The bowl can be covered with a plain, clear glass lid if you wish, but it is best not to cover it. If debris enters the water, skim it off with a clear crystal or with your washed hands at the end of the process. Pour the essence into the glass bottles and remove the gemstone. When handling more than one gemstone essence, wash your hands between them to prevent one coming in contact with the other.

Do this process and handle the gemstones, bowls and elixirs only when in a positive frame of mind, preferably in a meditative state. Your vibrations enter the elixirs, too. To completely neutralize the remedies from your emotions or any vibrations held in the gemstones, set the filled bottles under a copper pyramid for half to two hours. This also helps to potentize them. The energy of the sun on the cleared stone and almost sterile water is the potentizing factor. Moonlight works also, especially for moon-oriented gemstone energies, and on the night of the full moon. These bottles of potentized essence are called the mother tincture.

Elixirs can be prepared with brandy instead of distilled water, but unlike the flower remedies and homeopathics, water is preferred. Gem elixirs can also be made homeopathically, placing the stone in alcohol (vodka or brandy) and making a tincture of it, then using one drop of the mother tincture to nine or ninety-nine drops of alcohol and succussing it (shaking it vigorously fifteen to twenty times). This is a 1x or 1c remedy, and the process is repeated to the desired potency. Another method of making a gemstone elixir is to boil the gem in a glass pot of distilled water, preferably at sunrise, noon or a full moon night. Remedies made on the wiccan Sabbats would be even more powerful. Place boiled essences under a pyramid for further potentizing, but the sun method is still the best one.

If the elixir is made homeopathically, place drops of the potentized and succussed mixture on milk sugar globules or tablets, and take them by placing the tablets under the tongue. If used as a liquid (sun-made or homeopathically prepared), a stock bottle can be used, placing seven drops of the mother tincture in an eyedropper bottle of pure water; like flower remedies, the mother tincture can also be used undiluted. Use the stock bottle in the same way as for flower remedies. Place drops of the essence (three, five or seven are magical numbers) under the tongue about four times a day, on waking, before bed, and between but not close to meals. They can be used more frequently in acute healing issues. Use one elixir for about a month and then reevaluate, but it is seldom positive to use the same elixir for longer than a year. The process above could be used to make flower remedies at home, as well as gemstone essences. A homeopathically made gemstone essence can be started from the sun method, as homeopathic gem remedies are made by powdering the gemstone, while the sun method keeps the stone intact and is more powerful. As in other homeopathic remedies, it is primarily the astral imprint, rather than any physical component that becomes the essence used for healing.

Gemstone elixirs are highly sensitive to environment and vibrations and need to be stored carefully.[9] Keeping them under a pyramid or surrounded by crystals protects their energies. Odors effect them, as in homeopathic remedies, and camphor, peppermint or drinking coffee will damage or inactivate them. The remedies are best stored away from the kitchen. Like flower remedies and herbal tinctures, finished gem essences should not be exposed to sun, but kept in brown or blue glass bottles (blue is optimal) in a dark place away from sunlight. The bottles should not touch each other and should not be stored in plastic or plastic bags. Wipe the bottles periodically with sea salt and water on a linen or cotton cloth, and/or place them under a pyramid or in a ring of clear quartz crystals to purify and enhance them. Homeopathic remedies and flower remedies also benefit from time under a pyramid at intervals, and are kept there for twenty-four hours. If remedies touch each other in storage, their vibrations can be separated and purified by time under a pyramid.

Any gemstone can be made into an elixir, if a specimen of the raw stone is available to make it with. Choose the stones for their healing uses on specific issues, first by matching the chakra color and then going by the individual stone's abilities. A chart in chapter one designates the chakra and gemstone color for various healing issues. See *The Women's Book of Healing* for a variety of gemstones and their individual uses, and use that to guide your gemstone choice. A few gemstones not covered in *The Women's Book of Healing* are given here with their indications.

Beginning with the root center, **hematite** is attracting increasing attention, and many women who see it in my workshops are drawn to this shiny, black, metallic stone. The energy is a stress releaser and potent grounder. This is the stone that runs red when cut, and is used to stop bleeding and prevent hemorrhaging. Black on the outside and red within, it is the inside and outside of the womb and used in childbirth. The stone eases worry and the mental treadmill described in the White Chestnut flower remedy, and lessens heavy menstrual flows. It's a gemstone and elixir for mental achievement and original thinking, and a fever-reducing agent.[10]

Elestials are a form of heat-blackened quartz, naturally etched and carved on their surfaces in an interesting and unique way. They are root center and crown center gemstones, not easy to find and expensive, but highly powerful for healing. In laying on of stones, they are used to open chakra blocks and forge awareness. Elestials in elixir help women assimilate karma for better grounding on the earth plane, as well as activating the crown and third eye spirituality levels. They help mental confusion and confused thought-form patterns, stabilize brainwaves, and are a source for tapping universal knowledge from within. They work deeply to discover the source in emotional healing issues and to help in transformation. Elestials also help and comfort women approaching death in terminal illness, easing the fear of dying.[11]

Red/orange gemstones in elixirs include red quartz and red

phantom quartz. **Red phantom quartz** is a clear quartz crystal containing a fuzzy-looking reddish inclusion that mirrors the crystal shape but is inside it. The points are usually small, around an inch long, and are becoming easier to locate. In laying on of stones or in a gem elixir this odd-looking crystal is positive for helping to release angers held inside. Where internalized anger and frustrations are held so tightly within that they cause physical dis-ease, as in arthritis, an elixir of this gemstone or its use in healing is helpful and positive. The red/orange gemstones are used for root and belly chakra dis-eases, often overlapping.

Red quartz is a crystalline, opaque form of quartz crystal that is brick red in color. It is an activator of the belly chakra, and positive for stimulating energy. Use it for AIDS, uterine, ovarian or fallopian tube dis-eases and cysts, for infertility, endometriosis, arthritis, asthma and allergies. It brings on menses and increases flow, and stimulates warmth and heat. Some women with menstrual problems find help with it. The stone is not a frequent one to locate, but is beginning to be more available. A small crystal is very powerful for elixirs.

For the solar plexus center, **sunstone** is a transparent golden gem found in Oregon. While suffering from the flu I used it to help with nausea, and it has a wonderfully cleansing and lemony astringent feeling. Sunstone is an elixir remedy for women with chronic sore throats or tonsillitis, and for athelete's cartilage issues. It's good for vitality and tension, especially the pit-of-the-stomach type of tension, for rheumatism, tired feet and spinal problems. It's a mood brightener and dispels fear.[12]

Golden or **amber calcite** is another solar plexus energy, a very gentle one. It's a mental stimulant, bringing spiritual levels of thought to manifest creatively, a good energy for students, writers or teachers. Calcite helps with astral projection and aids the woman to remember where she has been when astral traveling. It balances and stimulates the pancreas, kidneys and spleen, helping to clear the body of toxins, and balances the inner yin and yang. Like sunstone, calcite is a fear-dispeller and mood-raiser.[13] It's energizing but less wiring than many solar plexus stones.

Heart center gemstones and elixirs include chrysoprase and dioptase for green gemstones and kunzite for a rose one. **Kunzite** is a lovely pink-lavender crystalline gem resembling tourmaline, one of the gentlest and most positive energies I have found. It is used for healing issues of the cardiovascular system, for the eyes, kidneys, and lower back issues. The stone contains lithium, a major element used in treatment of manic-depressive dis-ease. Kunzite is also positive for such dis-eases as alcoholism, anorexia, arthritis, epilepsy, headaches, Meniere's dis-ease, thyroid issues, phobias, memory loss, colitis, mental illness and schizophrenia. It is considered a help in aplastic anemia. The stone is an emotional regenerator, used for self-esteem issues and for stabilizing emotions and moods. It's a lovely calmative in stress or emotional pain.[14]

Chrysoprase is an apple green heart center gemstone, used for emotional and physical balance. Definitely a Cancer sign gem, this is a flowing energy that helps a woman to see both sides of an issue and to flow with changes. It enhances sensitivity on all levels, including artistic sensitivity. Physically the energy is for eye problems, gout and to ease emotional upsets. It raises depression and is especially powerful for all aspects of infertility in women.[15] This is an interesting and beautiful stone that women need to take more notice of.

Dioptase is another green heart center gemstone, this time of a dark metallic green. Its energy is for prosperity, nourishment and well-being, and it's used to relieve poverty of the body, mind or spirit. Physically, dioptase is used for headaches, migraines, surgical afterpain, and any sort of pain; it eases high blood pressure and stress issues, and expands consciousness of sources of dis-ease.[16]

Throat center gemstones are light blue, and sometimes blue/green stones that bridge the heart and throat centers. Once heart center issues are opened they are released through the throat center, and issues of one chakra are often linked to the other center as well. **Chrysocolla** has long been my favorite gemstone, and particularly the soft form (rather than gem silica) works well in a gemstone elixir. Any issue of the cardiovascular system is helped by this energy, high blood pressure, migraines, lung issues, lethargy and stress. The stone is a thought amplifier, a physical and creativity stimulant, an opener and balancer of the heart and throat centers. It reduces fear, guilt, tension, ulcers, digestive problems, hypoglycemia, asthma and decalcifies the joints in arthritis. It's a mood-raiser and many women with menstrual difficulties benefit from it. Musicians and writers especially like this bright aqua gem. This is a feminine/lunar gemstone energy that is an all-healer.[17]

A woman asked me to include **Amazonite** in this section and to tell women of its importance in sobriety. Several women I know are using it successfully for this. The energy is a soother of the entire nervous system, balancing the solar plexus, heart and throat. The stone helps in balancing calcium, osteoporosis, tooth decay, muscle spasms and twitching. It is helpful wherever a muscle relaxant is needed, including in epilepsy. Amazonite is a light aqua gemstone that soothes and balances all the chakras.[18]

Little or nothing has been written on blue topaz or celestite, but women in my workshops are very much drawn to these light blue stones and I am, too. **Celestite** is a delicate blue crystalline mineral, sometimes having tiny crystals on every side of it. The stone reflects a peace and purity that is very clear, very gentle and positive. To hold a piece of celestite is to become still inside, and to feel as clear and pure as a mountain stream. It generates a coolness, peace and flowing. In an elixir, try this gem to calm the mind, ease worrying thoughts and stress, for meditation and psychic healing work, headaches and migraines, and to loosen rigidity to an easy flow. This is a mental, emotional and spiritual relaxant and a mood-raiser. The stone's color suggests spirituality and creativity.

Blue topaz is a translucent light blue stone, varying in the amount of blue included in it, and sometimes containing rainbows. The bluer the specimen, the more powerful. I wear a blue topaz for releasing anger, and sometimes it stimulates more release than is comfortable. This is a stone for migraines and stress headaches, for sore throats that come from holding in what you need to say. By closing the throat, women prevent themselves from saying things that could be a danger to them, but unless the emotions and anger are released dis-ease develops. Use an elixir of blue topaz to release a blocked throat chakra and open the anger safely.

Gemstone elixirs for the brow chakra include kyanite, azurite and iolite. **Kyanite** is a light blue-silver, almost metallic gemstone with fibers running longways through it. The stone splits and splinters along these fibers, but is otherwise surprisingly strong. I have carried a piece in my much-battered pockets for more than a year now, with it not being much damaged. Kyanite is from Montana and quite inexpensive. Many women are drawn to it. The stone is a gentle all-chakra balancer and calmative that helps in releasing angers and frustrations. It's positive in meditation and insomnia, headaches and migraines, and has a feminine/lunar third eye opening energy.[19] Because of its light color, some crystal women would class this stone with the throat center, and it has throat chakra uses. But I feel it to be a third eye gemstone for its meditative and psychic/clairvoyance uses and urge women to work more with it.

Azurite is a very deep indigo color, the color most associated with the brow chakra, and has an astringent, penetrating quality. It dissolves negative thoughts, is a powerful psychic opener, and is an energy for looking deep within (whether content with what you see or needing to change it). This gemstone energy amplifies creativity, psychic ability and healing skill, femininity and consciousness. Use it in meditation and healing work, and to clear the etheric double and mental bodies. Physical uses include bone dis-eases, arthritis, inflammations, inflamed skin issues, spinal curvature, hypothyroidism, lymphatic issues and multiple sclerosis. This elixir increases assimilation of zinc and other minerals.[20]

Iolite is a violet/indigo gemstone that is very positive for women drawn to it. This is a beautiful translucent to opaque stone, a third eye opener and crown chakra balancer, a bridge energy between the two centers. The stone and elixir are useful for women learning to channel and women first opening to spirituality/Goddess consciousness. It connects women with their Goddess-within and is a help for those just opening psychically who might be frightened by that process. The stone is a gentle stabilizer and awareness opener that needs more women's notice and analysis.

Phantom quartz is a greyish-opaque form of quartz crystal, not especially attractive when found tumbled. Images seem to move around inside it. (This is not the same stone as quartz phantoms, crystals with the images of other crystals inside them.) The stone is highly positive for women doing past life regression work and delving into issues that need visualizing and solving. Taking it to bed one night, I began to see a running film of images of happenings moving further and further into the past. Like other opaque/white brow-to-crown bridging stones, the images were of things that needed looking at, but that I had been avoiding. Aragonite also has this quality of forcing one to resolve issues. A woman who used phantom quartz for past life regression work was delighted with it. The images from it are sharp and clear, and highly defined for place and time. Take this elixir in small doses, the third eye/crown white gemstones can be harsh.

In gemstones and elixirs for the crown center, **sugulite** (also called luvulite or royal azel), is a new gem rediscovered recently in the Kalahari desert of South Africa. Its color is a reddish-violet with sometimes black lines running through, and is a root/crown connecting energy. Katrina Raphaell credits it with releasing pressures and stresses as a cancer preventive. It's a protective energy that helps women integrate their spirituality into daily life. The gem or elixir is a good one for aware, sensitive, idealistic women who have difficulty accepting evil in the world.[21] It is also useful to women who need help integrating their right and left brain hemispheres—dyslexics, epileptics, women with physical coordination or vision problems, and women with motor skill or nerve issues. Sugulite opens and balances the crown and third eye centers, and helps women to mature spiritually.[22] I found carrying a piece of this gemstone to be very centering, but its high price out of line. Considering the political situation in South Africa, many women will choose not to wear it. It also comes from Japan, but the pieces I have seen are all from Africa.

Lepidolite is another violet gemstone for the crown chakra, containing many of the same properties as kunzite, though kunzite is more heart-focused. The stone is a sparkly, powdery material, soft and metallic-specked and often containing inclusions of rubellite (pink tourmaline) that connects it to the heart. Lepidolite contains a high content of lithium, and is a nervous system calmative positive for all the dis-eases that kunzite helps. There is more spirituality/crown chakra orientation to lepidolite, as compared to kunzite. The energy is calming and stabilizing to the mind, emotions and central nervous system. It's an aid to digestion and to metabolizing calcium in the body. An elixir of this energy reduces stress and raises depression. It connects the cycle of birth and death, helping the transition into or out of life for infants and elders.[23] I have seen it combined with mica in a silvery-purple sheet that is beautiful and highly positive for meditation work.

Gemstone elixirs for the transpersonal point include clear quartz crystal and herkimer diamonds. **Herkimer diamonds** are balancers of the physical with the spiritual. They are helpful for mental or emotional imbalance, bring harmony between two women, and are meditation enhancers. This stone as an elixir reduces and releases stress and tension, and detoxifies the body.[24]

Clear quartz crystal as an essence or elixir removes negative thought-forms and thought-patterns, raises spirituality and consciousness, increases psychic ability, focuses meditation and enhances all forms of healing. Clear crystal is a balancer and amplifier of all energies and is positive used with any other gem essence or gemstone. It balances the body, emotions, mind and spirit, aiding in all functions of the body and of the aura bodies. The stone is the essence of yin/feminine/Goddess energy and eases all dis-ease states.[25] Any woman who has worked with clear crystal knows a thousand healing uses for it. Make sure the stone is fully cleared before making it into an elixir.

Women who use gemstones and crystals for laying on of stones or other healing will appreciate their abilities in gemstone elixirs. Like flower remedies, gem elixirs create positive changes in women's auras over a period of time. The changes come gently and sometimes imperceptibly, but they come. More and more women are working with these. I would like to warn, however, against being 'taken' by prepared essences at high prices. The stones can be made into elixers at home with a minimum of expense and equipment, and it is not necessary or positive to spend thirty dollars, as one women did, for a bottle of 'magickal crystal essence.' Another thing to note in the making of gemstone elixers is the optional use of a pyramid. Pyramids can be made at home of anything from cardboard to copper tubing and are important means for clearing stones and altar tools, for preserving and detoxifying. A friend has a six-foot pyramid to sleep under and it's wonderful; it's a calmative, balancer and healer. This is another tool new to women, probably from Atlantis, and worth exploring.

NOTES

1. Malcolm Hulke, Ed., *The Encyclopedia of Alternative Medicine and Self-Help*, (New York, Schocken Books, 1979), p. 77.

2. Mechthild Scheffer, *Bach Flower Therapy, Theory and Practice*, (Rochester, VT, Thorsen's Publishing Group, 1986), p.18.

3. *Ibid.*, p. 207.

4. *Ibid.*, pp. 212–214.

5. Edward Bach, *The Twelve Healers and Other Remedies*, in *The Bach Flower Remedies*, (New Canaan, CT, Keats Publishing, 1977), p. 90. Definitions for the remedies come from here, and from Mechthild Scheffer, *Bach Flower Therapy*, as well as Bach Center USA, *The Bach Flower Remedies*.

6. Mechthild Scheffer, *Bach Flower Therapy*, p. 204.

7. *Ibid.*, p. 205.

8. The process is described in Gurudas, *Gem Elixers and Vibrational Healing*, Vol. I, (Boulder, CO, Cassandra Press, 1985), pp. 23–27.

9. *Ibid.*, pp. 29–30.

10. Roger Calverley, *The Language of Crystals*, (Toronto, Radionics Research Association, 1986), p. 98. This is a very overpriced book but still worth the money.

11. Katrina Raphaell, *Crystal Healing*, (New York, Aurora Press, 1987), pp. 131–133. Katrina Raphaell's books are highly recommended.

12. Roger Calverley, *The Language of Crystals*, p. 132.

13. Katrina Raphaell, *Crystal Healing*, p. 192, and Gurudas, *Gem Elixirs and Vibrational Healing*, p. 88.

14. Gurudas, *Gem Elixirs and Vibrational Healing*, p. 121.

15. *Ibid.*, p. 91, and Roger Calverley, *The Language of Crystals*, p. 84.

16. Roger Calverley, *The Language of Crystals*, p. 86.

17. *Ibid.*, p. 82, and Gurudas, *Gem Elixirs and Vibrational Healing*, pp. 90-91.

18. Roger Calverley, *The Language of Crystals*, p. 68.

19. *Ibid.*, p. 104.

20. Gurudas, *Gem Elixirs and Vibrational Healing*, p. 82.

21 Katrina Raphaell, *Crystal Enlightenment*, (New York, Aurora Press, 1985), pp. 121–123.

22. Gurudas, *Gem Elixirs and Vibrational Healing*, p. 151.

23. Roger Calverley, *The Language of Crystals*, pp. 108–110.

24. *Ibid.*, p. 44, and Gurudas, *Gem Elixirs and Vibrational Healing*, pp. 114–115.

25. Gurudas, *Gem Elixirs and Vibrational Healing*, pp. 148–149.

Afterword

This book has been an introduction to many forms of women's healing, some familiar and others not, but all going back to early women's healing and probably to the matriarchies. The woman who begins the road as a healer takes many paths, and she follows where her interests and intuitions lead her. All the ways of women's healing are positive and have much to offer those who participate in them, either for self-healing or for healing and helping others. The modern medical system is too often negative for women, with a few exceptions of some caring female physicians who are open to nontraditional ways. Self-help that heals a dis-ease before it gets serious enough for medical care helps to avoid the drugs and surgeries that are traumatic, expensive and often worsen the dis-ease. I hope in time that healing and medicine can join forces, adding the best and most positive of medical technology to the non-invasive, gynocentric and respectful attitudes of women's healing. Until that day, we do it ourselves as much as possible, taking our own power and control.

A comment from my friend Nett Hart, is appropriate here:

> I think we also have to acknowledge that many of the diseases we have today were not known in the times of the women healers. A toxic environment, radiation, stress, accidents with machinery and cars, VDTs, radio waves and short waves, food additives/chemicals, substance abuse—all create dis-ease concomitant with the technologies with which they are often treated. Health is not an individual cause, but a responsibility we all share to stop the spoilage of the earth and the wasting of her creatures. Until that happens, those most oppressed by this patriarchal system will be further disadvantaged by its diseases and the expense of treatment.

As daughters of the line of women healers, a line extending from the matriarchies to today, we have our work cut out for us.

Women learn healing through books, workshops, dialogue with other healers, and from going to Goddess-within to experiment and find what works. Most of my own healing has come from book research and from trying the methods myself, before recommending them to others. Any form of women's networking is helpful and valuable in healing. This book is a compilation of self-help, group work and healing theory. The material is derived by research and use, and by learning from other women. For the woman using it, I suggest working with your own healing issues first, using the method or methods that interest and attract you, before branching out to helping others. If a subject interests you particularly, read the books referenced for it and go further. No one chapter can cover any healing method well.

For my sister who is a healer or becoming one, I wish you sincerest blessings. You are much needed by women in this world to heal the scars of patriarchy, racism, sexism, ageism, incest and ablism—and all the other isms. You are needed by the Goddess Earth to heal her as the Age of Pisces/patriarchy ends. I leave you with a phrase from the Chinese *I Ching* or *Book of Changes*, 'perseverance furthers,' and wish you the strength, light and clarity to continue.

When the spiritual powers are passed on and transmitted they can no longer turn back; and when they turn back they cannot be transmitted, and then their moving powers are lost to the universe. In order to fulfill destiny women should go beyond that which is near at hand and consider it as trifling. One should make public upon tablets of jade that which was hidden and concealed in treasuries and storehouses, to study it from early dawn until night, and thus make known the precious mechanism of the universe.

The Chinese *Nei Jing*, Fourth Century BCE

Resources

For more information on the subjects of this book or classes, send a stamped self-addressed envelope with inquiries.

Goddess Newsletter and Networking:
Of A Like Mind
POB 6021
Madison, WI 53716

Goddess Correspondence Course for Women:
Shekinah Mountainwater
POB 2991
Santa Cruz, CA 95063

The Aura:
The Theosophical Society of America
306 W. Geneva Rd.
Wheaton, IL 60187

Laying on of Stones:
Katrina Raphaell
Crystal Enlightenment
POB 3208
Taos, NM 87571

Diane Stein (workshops)
c/o The Crossing Press
POB 1048
Freedom, CA 95019

Reiki:
The American International Reiki Association, Inc.
POB 86038
St. Petersburg, FL 33738

Reiki Alliance
POB 5327
Eugene, OR 97505

American-International Reiki Association, Inc.
A.I.R.A.
2210 Wilshire Blvd, Suite 831
Santa Monica, CA 90403

The Radiance Technique Journal (Publication)
POB 8156
St. Petersburg, FL 33738

Polarity Balancing:
American Polarity Therapy Association
POB 19459
Seattle, WA 98109

International Polarity Foundation
511 Main St.
Fort Lee, NJ 07024

Shiatsu and Acupressure:
Wataru Ohashi
Shiatsu Education Center
52 W. 55 St.
New York, NY 10019

Pauline Sasaki
151A Scribner Ave.
Norwalk, CT 06854

Reflexology:
International Institute of Reflexology
POB 12642
St. Petersburg, FL 33733-2642

Reflexology Tools and Correspondence Course:
Stirling Enterprises, Inc.
POB 216
Cottage Grove, OR 97424

Applied Kinesiology:
International College of Applied Kinesiology
POB 680547
Park City, UT 84068

Touch for Health Foundation
1174 N. Lake Ave.
Pasadena, CA 91104

Herbs:
Billie Potts
L.F.R.
POB 158
Summit, NY 12175

Susun Weed
Wise Woman Center
POB 64
Woodstock, NY 12498

Frontier Cooperative Herbs
Box 69
Norway, IA 52318

Goldenseal
1917 Murray Ave.
Pittsburgh, PA 15217

Lhasa Karnak Herb Co.
2513 Telegraph Ave.
Berkeley, CA 94704

Nature's Herbs
281 Ellis St.
San Francisco, CA 94102

STAMPS Apothecary
33 Van Buren
Eureka Springs, ARK 72632

No Common Scents
King's Yard
Yellow Springs, OH 45387

World Wide Herbs, Ltd.
11 St. Catharines East
Montreal 129, Quebec
Canada

Herbs and Midwifery Correspondence Course:
Jeannine Parvati Baker
Hygieia College
POB 398
Monroe, UT 84754

Homeopathic Associations:
National Center for Homeopathy
1500 Massachusetts Ave. NW
Washington, DC 20005

International Foundation for Homeopathy
1141 NW Market St.
Seattle, WA 98107

Homeopathic Pharmacies:
Boericke and Tafel, Inc.
1011 Arch St.
Philadelphia, PA 19107

John A. Bornemann Co.
1208 Amosland Rd.
Norwood, PA 19074

Homeopathic Educational Services
2124 Kittredge St.
Berkeley, CA 94704

Standard Homeopathic Co.
POB 61067
Los Angeles, CA 90661

Luyties Pharmacal Co.
4200 Laclede Ave.
St. Louis, MO 63108

Erhart and Karl, Inc.
17 N. Wabash Ave.
Chicago, IL 60602

Washington Homeopathic Pharmacy
4914 Delray Ave.
Bethesda, MD 20814

Homeopaths:
Sidney Spinster Skinner
Nurse-Homeopath
Preventive Medicine Associates
10700 Old County Rd 15, Suite 350
Minneapolis, MN 55441

Bach Flower Remedies:
Ellon Bach USA, Inc.
644 Merrick Road
Lynnbrook, NY 11563

The Bach Centre
Mount Vernon
Sotwell
Wallingford
Oxon OX10 OPZ
England

Gemstone Elixers:
Gemstoned, Inc.
2 Waverly Place
New York, NY 10003

AIDS:
Project Inform
347 Dolores St., Suite 301
San Francisco, CA 94110
1-800-822-7422

No/AIDS Task Force
POB 2616
New Orleans, LA 70176

Women's AIDS Network
San Francisco AIDS Foundation
333 Valencia St. 4th Fl.
San Francisco, CA 94103

AIDS Action Committee
661 Boylston St., Suite 4
Boston, MA 02116

Hay House
3029 Wilshire Blvd., #206
Santa Monica, CA 90404

HEAL (Health Education AIDS Laison)
POB 60
New York, NY 10014

The Aliveness Project
c/o Steven Katz
5307 Russel S.
Minneapolis, MN 55410

Bibliography

Margot Adair. *Working Inside Out, Tools for Change.* Berkeley, CA, Wingbow Press, 1984.

Agency France Press. "Ancient Feminist Script Found in China." *Minnesota Star Tribune,* Sunday, May 18, 1986.

Frank Alper. *Exploring Atlantis,* Three Volumes. Phoenix, AZ, Metaphysical Society, 1982.

Jose Arguelles. *The Mayan Factor.* Sante Fe, NM, Bear and Co., 1987.

Suzanne Arms. *Immaculate Deception: A New Look at Women and Childbirth in America.* New York, Bantam Books, 1975.

Bach Centre USA. *The Bach Flower Remedies,* pamphlet. Windemere, NY, Bach Centre USA, 1983.

Edward Bach. "The Twelve Healers and Other Remedies." In *The Bach Flower Remedies.* New Canaan, CT, Keats Publishing, 1977.

Lawrence Badgley, MD. *Healing AIDS Naturally.* San Bruno, CA, Human Energy Press, 1987.

Cathryn Bauer. *Acupressure for Women.* Freedom, CA, The Crossing Press, 1987.

Beijing Medical College. *Dictionary of Chinese Traditional Medicine.* Hong Kong, Commercial Press, Ltd., 1984.

Biokinesiology Institute. *Muscle Testing: Your Way to Health.* Shady Cove, OR, Biokinesiology Institute, 1982.

Margery Blackie, MD. *The Patient, Not the Cure: The Challenge of Homeopathy.* Santa Barbara, CA, Woodbridge Press, 1976.

William Boericke, MD. *The Pocket Manual of Homeopathic Materia Medica with Repertory.* New Delhi, India, B. Jain Publishers Pvt., Ltd., 1984.

Catherine Bowman. *Crystal Awareness.* St. Paul, Llewellyn Publications, 1988.

Roger Calverley. *The Language of Crystals.* Toronto, Canada, Radionics Research Associates, 1986.

Mildred Carter. *Body Reflexology.* W. Nyack, NY, Parker Publishing Co., 1983.

Mildred Carter. *Hand Reflexology: Key to Perfect Health.* W. Nyack, NY, Parker Publishing Co., 1975.

Mildred Carter. *Helping Yourself With Foot Reflexology.* W. Nyack, NY, Parker Publishing Co., 1969.

Sandra Chase, MD. *Homeopathy, A Brief Overview.* Washington, DC, National Center for Homeopathy, 1981. (pamphlet).

Judy Chicago. *The Birth Project.* New York, Doubleday and Co., 1985.

Judy Chicago. *The Dinner Party, A Symbol of Our Heritage.* New York, Doubleday and Co., 1979.

Linda Clark. *Get Well Naturally.* New York, Arco Books, 1982.

Cobra. "Herbcraft: Remedies for Vaginitis." In *Goddess Rising,* (4006 1st NE, Seattle, WA 98103), Issue 20, Spring, 1988.

Stephen Cummings, FPN and Dana Ullman, MPH. *Everybody's Guide to Homeopathic Medicines.* Los Angeles, Jeremy Tarcher, Inc., 1984.

Mary Daly. *Websters' First Intergalactic Wickedary of the English Language.* Boston, Beacon Press, 1988.

Adele Davis. *Let's Get Well.* New York, Signet Books, 1965.

John Diamond, MD. *Your Body Doesn't Lie.* New York, Warner Books, 1979.

Hugh Drummond, MD. *Dr. Drummond's Spirited Guide to Health Care in a Dying Empire.* New York, Grove Press, 1980.

Barbara Ehrenreich and Dierdre English. *For Her Own Good: 150 Years of the Experts' Advice to Women.* New York, Anchor Books, 1979.

Barbara Ehrenreich and Dierdre English. *Witches, Midwives and Nurses: A History of Women Healers.* Old Westbury, NY, The Feminist Press, 1973.

Anya Fields. *Dowsing Dykes.* Milwaukee, WI, Crystal Revelations, 1982.

Marija Gimbutas. *The Goddesses and Gods of Old Europe: Myths and Cult Images.* Berkeley and Los Angeles, University of CA Press, 1974 and 1982.

Robert Gordon. *Your Healing Hands: The Polarity Experience.* Santa Cruz, CA, Unity Press, 1978.

Mrs. M. Grieve. *A Modern Herbal,* Two Volumes. New York, Dover Books, 1931.

Gurudas. *Gem Elixers and Vibrational Healing, Vol. I.* Boulder, Co, Cassandra Press, 1985.

Nett Hart and Lee Lanning. *Awakening: An Almanac of Lesbian Lore and Vision.* Minneapolis, Word Weavers, 1987.

Louise L. Hay. *The AIDS Book: Creating a Positive Approach.* Santa Monica, CA, Hay House, 1988.

Louise L. Hay. *You Can Heal Your Life.* Santa Monica, CA, Hay House, 1984.

David Hoffman. *The Holistic Herbal.* Scotland, The Findhorn Press, 1983.

Malcolm Hulke. *The Encyclopedia of Alternative Medicine and Self-Help.* New York, Schocken Books, 1979.

Mildred Jackson, ND and Terri Teague, ND, DC. *The Handbook of Alternatives to Chemical Medicine.* Berkeley, CA, Bookpeople, 1975.

Priscilla Kapel. *The Body Says Yes.* San Diego, CA, ACS Publications, 1981.

Ted Kaptchuk, OMD. *The Web That Has No Weaver: Understanding Chinese Medicine.* New York, Congdon and Weed, 1983.

Velma Keith and Monteen Gordon. *The How To Herb Book.* Pleasant Grove, UT, Mayfield Publishing Co., 1984.

Kathi Keville. "Strengthening Your Immune System with Herbs". In *Vegetarian Times*, July, 1985. Reprint.

Audre Lorde. "An Open Letter to Mary Daly." In Cherrie Moraga and Gloria Anzaldua, Eds. *This Bridge Called My Back: Writings by Radical Women of Color.* Watertown, MA, Persephone Press, 1981.

Lucinda Liddell. *The Book of Massage.* New York, Simon and Schuster, Inc., 1984.

George Meek. *Healers and the Healing Process.* Wheaton, IL, Quest/Theosophical Society Books, 1977.

John Meyer. *The Herbalist.* Glenwood, Il, Meyerbooks, 1918.

Earl Mindell. *The Vitamin Bible.* New York, Warner Books, 1985.

Paul David Mitchell. *The Usui System of Natural Healing.* Couer d'Alene, ID, The Reiki Alliance, 1985.

Muriel Nellis. *The Female Fix.* Boston, Houghton Mifflin Co., 1980.

Greg Nielsen and Joseph Polansky. *Pendulum Power.* Rochester, VT, Destiny Books, 1987.

Billie Potts. *Witches Heal: Lesbian Herbal Self-Sufficiency.* Bearsville, NY, Hecuba's Daughters Press, 1981.

Prevention Magazine Staff. *The Complete Book of Vitamins.* Emmaus, PA, Rodale Press, 1977.

Prevention Magazine Staff. *The Complete Book of Minerals For Health.* Emmaus, PA, Rodale Press, 1972.

Katrina Raphaell. *Crystal Healing.* New York, Aurora Press, 1987.

Katrina Raphaell. *Crystal Enlightenment.* New York, Aurora Press, 1985.

Barbara Ray, Ph.D. *The Reiki Factor.* St. Petersburg, FL, Radiance Associates, 1983.

John D. Rea. *Patterns of the Whole, Vol. I: Healing and Quartz Crystals.* Boulder, CO, Two Trees Publishing Co., 1986.

Harold Rosenberg, Ph.D. *The Book of Vitamin Therapy.* New York, Berkeley Books, 1974.

Mechthild Scheffer. *Bach Flower Therapy, Theory and Practice.* Rochester, VT, Thorsen's Publishing Group, 1986.

Barbara Seaman and Gideon Seaman, MD. *Women and the Crisis in Sex Hormones.* New York, Rawson Associates Publishers, Inc., 1977.

Maruti Seidman. *A Guide to Polarity Therapy.* N. Hollywood, CA. Newcastle Publishing Co., 1986.

Stephanie Matthews-Simonton, O. Carl Simonton, MD, and James L. Creighton. *Getting Well Again.* New York, Bantam Books, 1984, Original, 1978.

Phyllis Speight. *Homeopathic Remedies for Women's Ailments.* Great Britain, Health Science Press, 1985.

Diane Stein. *Stroking the Python: Women's Psychic Lives.* St. Paul, MN,

Llewellyn Publications, 1989.

Diane Stein. *The Women's Book of Healing.* St. Paul, Llewellyn Publications, 1988.

Diane Stein. *The Women's Spirituality Book.* St. Paul, Llewellyn Publications, 1987.

Diane Stein. *The Kwan Yin Book of Changes.* St. Paul, Llewellyn Publications, 1985.

Merlin Stone. *Ancient Mirrors of Womanhood: A Treasury of Goddess and Heroine Lore from Around the World.* Boston, Beacon Press, 1984.

Merlin Stone. *When God Was A Woman.* New York, Harcourt, Brace, Jovanovich, 1978.

Randolph Stone, DC, DO. *Polarity Balancing, Vol. I.* Reno, NV, CRCS Publications, 1986.

Lina G. Strauss. *Diseases in Milk.* New York, E.P. Dutton Co., 1917.

Iona Marsaa Teeguarden. *Acupressure Way of Health: Jin Shin Do.* New York, Japan Publications, 1978.

Robert Temple. *The Sirius Mystery.* Rochester, VT, Inner Traditions Intl. Ltd., 1987.

John Thie, DC. *Touch For Health.* Marina del Rey, CA, DeVorss and Co. Publishers, 1979.

Dana Ullman. *Homeopathy: Medicine for the 21st Century.* Berkeley, CA, N. Atlantic Books, 1988.

"Vital Vitamins." In *Light News*, (POB 770844, Houston, TX 72215), Vol. I, no. 3, March–April, 1988.

Frank Waters. *Book of the Hopi.* New York, Ballantine Books, 1963.

Tony Webb, Tim Lang and Kathleen Tucker. *Food Irradiation: Who Wants It?* Rochester, VT, Thorsens Publishing Group, 1987.

Susun Weed. *WiseWoman Herbal for the Childbearing Year.* Woodstock, NY, Ash Tree Publishing, 1985.

Index

Diane Stein

I was born on September 22, 1948 (Virgo Sun, Taurus Moon, Sag Rising) in Pittsburgh, PA and raised in Pittsburgh. Education includes a Bachelor of Science degree in Secondary Education/English from Duquesne University and a Master of Arts degree in English Literature from the University of Pittsburgh (1972). I have been writing seriously since high school and was assistant editor of the Duquesne University student literary magazine. In 1969 I began publishing in small press magazines and journals, including some of the earliest women's movement publications. I entered feminism from the anti-Vietnam movement, came out as a lesbian by 1972, and began writing Goddess poetry in 1977. I have never been in 'the closet' as a lesbian or witch.

I was introduced to wicce by books I read in high school and rejected for their male orientation, but when healing and the Goddess became connected to the women's movement, I joined it. At first it was a literary connection through women's herstory, politics and poetry. It became a religion and a coming home for me in 1982 when Starhawk's *The Spiral Dance* connected the Craft and Goddess to activism and psychic skills. I became a priestess quickly, first in writing and then in practice. I started learning healing and led my first ritual at the 1983 Michigan Women's Music Festival (the same week I attended my first ritual!) and have entered most facets of feminist wicce since. I had just begun *The Kwan Yin Book of Changes* that summer.

The Craft for me is activism in women's rights and a way of life. Though primarily a healer, I have worked politically in the lesbian and gay rights movements, the anti-war movement, and in the areas of AIDS, incest recovery and disability rights. I am differently abled with a curvature of the spine, visual impairments and dyslexia, and aware of disabled women's needs and strengths.

My primary interest in the Craft is in healing—learning it, practicing it and teaching it to others. I feel all women are healers, that it is our heritage and right, and that my role in this lifetime is to teach this concept and the methods to as many women as I can. When women learn to be healers they accept their own power and ability to heal themselves of the damage of living in a patriarchal world. When they have healed themselves they help others, and eventually work to heal the Earth herself. Most women need healing in some form at some time, and certainly the Goddess Earth does. I have devoted my life to learning as much as I can and teaching it in my books, workshops, individual healing sessions, and in the example of my own life. I devote my life to working with women.

At forty-two years old in 1990, I look forward to being a totally outrageous crone.

*The Crossing Press
publishes a full selection of
feminist titles.
To receive our current catalog,
please call —Toll Free—800/777-1048.*